IIFYM & FLEXIBLE DIETING COOKBOOK

Lose Weight and Build Muscles While Still Eating The Food You Love

Author

Mark Matthews

TABLE OF CONTENTS

Chapter 1

What is Macro?

Macros, short for macronutrients, are proteins, starches, and fats, the real supplements the body needs to work efficiently and proficiently, and the idea of tallying your macros is fundamentally ensuring that you get a particular measure of each in your day-by-day life by eating less carbs. Sugar—the sugars, starches, and filaments found in grains, organic products, and vegetables—have 4 calories for each gram. Protein, made up of corrosive amino chains basic for energizing the body also have 4 calories for every gram. Furthermore, fat is a higher-calorie macronutrient with 9 calories for every gram.

A full scale eating regimen takes the accentuation off calories and instead organizes the extent of proteins, fats and carbs, which are known as macros, hence the name.

Get the correct amounts of these nutrients and you'll become more fit, as well as be more successful at consuming fat and building slender muscles.

How about we examine each macronutrient to get an essential understanding of each.

Protein

Overview: Arguably the overlord in the realm of wellness nourishment, proteins are generally connected to building muscle and are essentially found in foods like meat and dairy. Be that as it may, its goes beyond muscles: it's the center segment for organs, bones, hair, compounds, and basically every kind of tissue in your body.

Proteins are made up of amino acids. Notwithstanding, there are 9 amino acids that are required for your body to work that your body can't synthesize itself. These are (appropriately) called essential amino acids, and the full 9 can be found from all meat sources. Shockingly for veggie lovers and vegetarians, it's uncommon to locate the full nine in vegetables and grains, so you have to ensure you eat a substantial assortment of foods in order to get all nine.

Starches

Overview: First companion then enemy, the food industry's association with starches has been whimsical to say the least. While it's actually the main macronutrient your body can get by without, doing so would be unpleasant. Carbs are your body's most effectively available wellspring of vitality, and is separated into glycogen (utilized by muscles) and glucose (utilized by the cerebrum).

Carbs can be partitioned into simple and complex starches. The two types allude to the length of the sugar particles. The shorter the atom chain is, the less demanding it is for your body to separate, so it's "easier"— they are essentially sugars. Then again, bigger particles such as starches, are "complex" since it takes more time for your body to separate it into usable segments.

In the realm of macros, a carb is a carb, regardless of whether it originates from sugars or starches. Let's be clear: this isn't an underwriting depending on Pop-Tarts and treats to meet your health goals. Actually, what you will see is that subsequent to checking macros for awhile, you'll presumably float towards complex wellsprings of carbs for satiety's sake. In any case, the opportunity for decision is there, and unwinding this limit amongst "great" and "awful" nourishments is essential to build up a more beneficial association with what you eat.

Fats

Overview: Fats are a key part of many diets. However, fat frequently gets unfavorable criticism since it's the most calorie-thick supplement out there. In any case, they're very important to your body, from the spine to vital hormone production it protects nerves, skin, hair, and so much more.

There are a bundle of various kinds of fats. Out of every one of them, the principle three you ought to be worried about are trans fats, omega-three unsaturated fats, and omega-six unsaturated fats.

Trans fats, informally known as "frankenfats," have been reliably shown to heighten the danger of coronary disease, and it ought to be stayed away from. They're typically found in pre-packaged foods and different brands of margarine.

The last two are what's known as fundamental unsaturated fats. Like fundamental amino acids, your body can't make them so you need to acquire them through your diet. Omega-3's can be found in fish, flax, and walnuts (take note of that they're all the more effectively assimilated from creature sources), and omega-6's from practically a wide range of oils.

It is totally obvious that it is a different eating regimens than that ones which marks certain foods as awful and even cut out whole nutrition types. The macro diet assumes that all kind of foods and nutrition types can be part of a diet.

This theory depends on the logical investigations that show that the quantity of food eaten is the most vital factor in losing or putting on weight. This is desirable over dodging or restricting a specific type of food.

Tallying macros actually offers a few nutritious advantages. For the dieting amateur, managing your dinner meals by tallying macros is a decent method to understand portion control. Additionally, it's absolutely adaptable for your personal objectives and body type, and it's flexible as indicated by the full-scale eating routine outcomes you're seeing (that's the reason it's additionally called adaptable abstaining from food).

What's more, it likewise shares some shared characteristics with Weight Watchers and calorie-checking in light of the fact that you do need to track your admission and remain inside specific ranges.

Be that as it may, it's not quite the same as other weight-control plans since it's not a one-type fits-all way of deal with counting calories.

In reality, one of the issues with conventional weight-control plans is that they don't take into account what you're eating, and the exact amount of calories you're consuming. Certainly, parcel control alone may work for some time, yet unless you change to the correct foods your discretion will change in the long run.

With a specific end goal in mind, it might be advantageous to center around macronutrients instead of calories. Some individuals do well on bring down starches and fats, while others on lowing their sugar intake. Making (and hitting) macronutrient targets enables you to figure out which works best for you, and at that point adhere to that sort of eating routine without expecting a total wipe out of either fat or sugars.

Chapter 2

The Basics of IIFYM

On the off chance that It Fits Your Macros, or IIFYM as the "cool kids" call it, is moderately new as a brand, the dietary standards have really been around for a long time in the weight training world, just under another name (macro diet).

IIFYM is an approach that spins around meeting daily macronutritional consumption targets, and not on what you eat to get there.

How about we see what it is precisely IIFYM ordered:

1. At the point when first beginning this diet you have to ascertain the correct number of macros that you need to achieve every day. You can do this by utilizing an online adding machine which figures the quantity of calories and measure of protein, starches, and fats you'll require for the day. The online number-cruncher considers how physically dynamic you are, your weight, stature, and your objectives. You can discover such a number cruncher on iifym.com When you figure out your macros you'll see just how adaptable you can be.

2. When you do that, the next activity is get yourself a journal and monitor all that you eat, measuring the nutrients you're

eating to ensure you're not gorging. Keeping a journal will show you the sorts of sustenance you can eat to achieve your full-scale objectives and you can likewise quantify the amounts with nourishment scales or different and versatile online applications.

One such application is "My Fitness Pal" where you can look at a huge database for incalculable nourishment items, even restaurant meals. It's adaptable, you can enter your own nourishments and there's likewise a standardized identification choice which will naturally enter the calories and macros of the item you examined. Studies have demonstrated that individuals who track their food intake tend to diminish their caloric intake intuitively.

3. IIFYM won't compel you to eat clean food, it'll enable you to eat food regarded as "not so perfect," and it will dependably keep you responsible so you don't go over your caloric objectives. Furthermore, it's not tied in with having the capacity to eat junk food as much. It's generally about finding the correct adjustment, and making a path toward abstaining from food more sustainable in the long haul.

As we stated, a few people contemplate eating junk food to achieve their large scale objectives; it's tied in with eating the food you like but with some restraint. IIFYM likewise enables you to scan for new nourishment decisions and enable you to achieve your wellness objectives by following the 80/20 rule. This implies getting 80% of your every day calories from natural, whole foods and the other 20% from treats.

Discover The Calories You Need

The quantity of calories you require every day is a result of your age, sex, weight, bulk, and action level. Eating more than this will make you put on weight, while eating less will help you shed pounds.

To make sense of the correct number you can utilize a calorie adding machine, but be careful as these have a tendency to be harsh gauges as they don't consider a bundle of elements that influence health, such as muscle to fat ratio or particular day-to-day exercise.

The best strategy is track what you typically eat for about seven days. Given that you aren't putting on weight or getting thinner, this would give you a smart thought to your every day calorie prerequisites.

For a direct route to weight reduction—that is around one pound for every week, you ought to make a calorie deficiency 500 calories for each day.

Calories and Macronutrients

There are two approaches to decide your macronutrient targets. The most straightforward technique is to distribute calories towards every supplement as indicated by a rate split. The most widely recognized split is 40:40:20, i.e. 40% of your calories allotted to protein, 40% to starches, and 20% to fats.

From there, working out what number of grams for each macronutrient you require involves basic math. For instance, say your objective caloric intake is 2,000 calories per day. You choose to part your macros as per a 40:40:20 split. From that point, utilize the accompanying counts:

Sugars

40% of your calories are given to your sugar admission.

2000 x 0.4 = 800 calories.

There are 4 calories/gram of carbs, so the aggregate sum is 200 grams of starches (800÷4=200).

Rehash this system for protein and fats.

Other prominent rate parts are 33:33:33 (an even measure of calories from each macronutrient) and 40:30:30 (40% protein, 30% sugars, 30% fat).

The adaptable eating regimen recommends an individual large scale objective that depends on your REE (resting vitality use).

This is joined with your day-by-day movement to shape up your TDEE (this adds up to every day vitality use).

To lose fat, expend less macros than your body requires. This is typically set at 20% relying upon what the individual's unique objectives are. By just advancing a direct calorie shortage will probably have gradual progression in the long term. This is superior to any fast weight reduction.

Once your TDEE and full scale proportions are resolved, you then count macros in the foods you eat. You continue to eat until the point that your large-scale objectives have been met for the day.

An illustration: Let's say that a woman's TDEE is 1,650 calories on her activity day. Those calories are then separated among the three macros at the accompanying rates:

- Protein: 30%

- Carbs: 45%

- Fat: 25%

As there are 4 calories for every gram of protein and sugars and 9 calories for every gram of fat, this converts into the accompanying amounts:

- Protein: 124 grams

- Carbs: 186 grams

- Fat: 46 grams

She then eats until the point that she hits every one of those objectives.

Is IIFYM ideal for you?

Full scale checking is most appropriate for objective-situated individuals. The individuals who have a reasonable vision of what they need to escape themselves may observe this to be the most effective way. For the individuals who will adhere to an arrangement, input a couple of numbers into a spreadsheet several times a day.

The individuals who are searching for a spotless, sound way of life aren't occupied with putting excessive time or intellectual prowess into it might be more joyful with a less complex calorie-counting system.

IIFYM, full scale tallying, abundant spreadsheets—whatever you call it—gets results. In any case, it's not the only method to advance. Regardless of whether this ends up being appropriate for you or not, don't make due with not as much as you need.

1. Mix it up. While tallying your macros doesn't really mean removing anything, there is an inclination to eat similar foods (like flame broiled chicken, dark rice, oats) over and over again. Likewise, you would prefer not to totally hold back on critical micronutrients, vitamins, or minerals on the grounds that your body requires them in lesser amounts. Stock up on nourishments high in cancer prevention agents (like berries) and essential vitamins and minerals (like verdant greens, dairy items, and splendid hued veggies) to ensure you're filling in your eating routine with the micronutrients that your body needs. On the off chance that despite everything you feel slow or off your amusement, consult your specialist or nutritionist.

2. Eat the correct sort of macronutrients. Not all fats or sugars are equal. The exact opposite thing you need to do is eat the greater part of your starches, including sugar (which Applegate says you should strive for 50 grams every day). With regards to fats, search for solid, unsaturated assortments like those in olive oil and nuts. You can also go for two servings a week of fish, such as salmon, to get in fundamental omega-3 fatty acids and all the flavor.

3. Don't scam yourself. Some large scales have their proportions off, rounding up when counting protein and carbs. While eating less carbs may influence you to think "weight reduction," you're really doing your body a noteworthy insult. "You require carbs in your eating routine, particularly in case you're more dynamic," says Applegate. In case you're not eating enough starches to fuel your hardest exercises, your body will begin to utilize the proteins in your muscles as fuel, rather than what it's implied for: to remake and repair muscles after action. At that point when protein is utilized as fuel, your muscles may wind up powerless, and development and reconstruction (read: muscle building and recuperation) will be traded off.

4. Get in contact with a health expert. Converse with a specialist or nutritionist before making a plunge. They can enable you to set shrewd, safe objectives, and even tip you off to where your objectives ought to be, given what your objectives are. Perhaps you're wanting to get thinner, pick up muscle, or basically keep up what you have going on. Whatever your objective may be, a specialist can ensure you're getting the fuel you require in the correct amounts.

Chapter 3

Whatever you want... not exactly!

The reality of the matter is that health food nuts can eat ANYTHING, however, only as long as it fits their recommended set of macros. This is great for some, for those who are originating from most diets that are extremely prohibitive.

It's the run-of-the-mill reaction of clean eaters, calorie counters, and the old school bad-to-the-bone muscle heads who assert that adaptable consumption of less calories doesn't work in any way, shape, or form.

They have this false belief that IIFYM is tied in with eating as much junk food as you can.

That isn't the situation by means.

Truth be told, it's truly far away from what most adaptable health food nuts really do, yet the myth still sustains itself that us in the IIFYM camp fill our day-by-day calories with chocolate, cake, pretzels, pizza, and doughnuts.

Of course, we do eat some foods that the overall population would consider "garbage," for a large portion of us, this really constitutes a little piece of our general eating regimen.

The question, however, still remains:

DOES THIS MEANS THAT JUNK FOOD IS ALLOWED?

While the adaptable eating regimen is more worried about the measure of nourishment, as opposed to how the sustenance is ordered, it recognizes the significance of practicing good eating habits.

Most backers of this eating style say that solid, whole foods ought to contain 78-84% of one's eating regimen, while 18-14% can be held out for foods marked as "garbage." This is a subjective term, yet things like chocolate, potatoes chips, french fries, and frozen yogurt would for the most part fall into this classification.

Adaptable calorie counters ought to likewise be aware of their fiber consumption. This guarantees that they are eating enough solid foods.

Ladies ought to make progress in excess of 25 grams for every day and men for at least 35 grams for each day. This is subject to your weight and age.

In case you're searching for a weight reduction arrangement that offers adaptability and plenty of nourishment decisions, then the adaptable eating regimen might be appropriate for you.

Do not worry if on a couple of days you are over one of your macros or under some others. It won't "destroy" your diet.

The most important thing as I see it is to hit as close to your TDEE as could be reasonably expected.

Macros are more for "calibrating" your outcomes, while your TDEE decides if you lose, keep up, or pick up.

So yes, work to meet your macros as these will enable you to achieve your objectives to the extent your body is concerned, yet eating 20 additional grams of fat on a specific day won't wreck your progress unless it puts you 180 calories over your TDEE.

On the off chance that you need a general rule, adhere to the 80:20 rule.

80% of your calories should be solid and full of nourishment, while 20% can originate from foods that you may classify as garbage.

Once more, this can differ upon your objectives and targets.

In case you're bodybuilding and need to get those calories in, I don't see an issue with going to 30% of junk food. Despite everything, you'll have the capacity to get enough fiber, vitamins, and minerals in, and increasing your junk food stipend makes it less demanding to hit your numbers.

When cutting calories however, 10% may do it, as increasing your healthy foods to 90% will keep you feeling considerably more full and satisfied.

The main issue, as usual, is to do what works for you and what you appreciate, then you can meet your goals and obtain positive outcomes.

Chapter 4

How to Track your Macros

When you know the amount of every macro to eat, you can start following your progress by utilizing a sustenance log.

Fortunately, this monotonous procedure is significantly less demanding then utilizing applications that offer expansive wholesome databases to monitor everything for you. Here are a couple to consider:

MyFitnessPal

MacroTracker

MyMacros+

MyNetDiary

Look for the nourishment you are eating in the application's database, alter the serving size and weight, and then click "done." The application will keep a running account of your macros as you eat for the duration of the day.

You'll additionally require a digital food scale.

This is to measure the bits of new nourishment like vegetables and meat since their health information is related to the weight of the specific sustenance. The scales are anything but difficult to use, and it makes for additional progression during the time spent.

You might need to design dinners so that you can similarly appropriate macros throughout the day.

You can simply wing it, yet in some cases you're left with couple of decisions towards the day's end.

For instance, in the event that you hit your fat and carb goals and have protein left, you'll need to pick nourishments like ultra-lean meats or whey protein with a specific end goal to then hit your protein target.

Allow me to give you an example of how to begin your weight reduction travel today:

- Purchase an advanced sustenance scale (measure your nourishment in grams, not cooked).

- Join to MyMacros+ (log the greater part of your nourishment in grams, not cooked).

- Utilize an IIFYM Calculator to get your correct fat macros in view of your particular body and vitality levels.

- Weigh all that you eat for the initial three months (in the long run you can eyeball it, however, we propose remaining steady with the scale for best outcomes) .

- Log each and every thing you eat, no matter how little or how "solid" you think it is. Always track what you eat!

- If dieting to lose fat, eat between 10% – 15% calories less than your body needs. If you are trying to bulk up, eat 12% more calories than your TDEE, every day (preferably from carbs)

- To dial in on an IIFYM with more precision, try these methods:

- Eat no less than .9 gram of protein for every pound of slender body weight (add up the body weight, less aggregate fat weight).

- Take between .2 – .3 grams of fat for every pound of slender body weight.

- Any residual calories you have left in your day-by-day accounting will originate from carbs

- Take in 15-20% of your slender body weight (in grams) of fiber consistently (this ought to be incorporated into your sugar intake).

- Drink 2 liters of water for every day, not including the other fluids you consume.

CHAPTER 5

50 IIFYM Recipes (Breakfast, Lunch, Snack, Dinner, Dessert)

BREAKFAST 1

RASPBERRY CHHIA PUDDING

NUTRITIONAL VALUE 342 Cal PROTEIN 9g FAT 24.9g
CARBOHYDRATES 11.4g

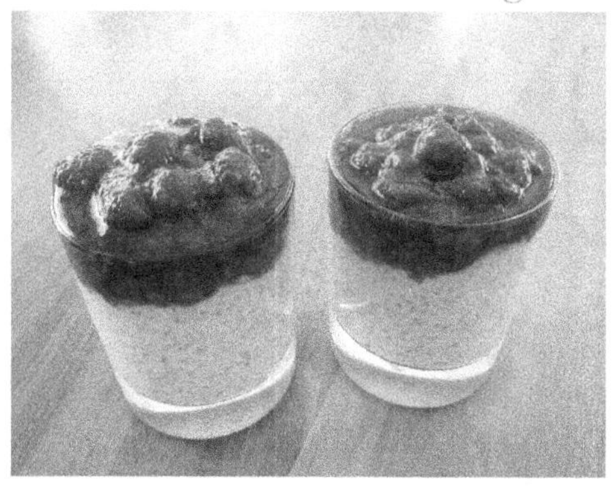

No matter if you are a vegan or a Paleo, dates could be your sweet respite. Check out this paleo chhia pudding that blends the dates flawlessly into the vanilla extract and coconut milk. Soft and warm, this raspberry paleo chhia pudding simply makes a delicious breakfast. Perfect for an occasional indulgence, they take some time to prepare, but worthy of the effort.

SERVES 5 PREPARATION TIME 15 MINUTES COOKING TIME
15 MINUTES

**6 pitted and quartered dates
1 - 12ounce can of coconut milk
1 ½ tbsp vanilla extract
1- 10 ounce of thawed and packaged raspberries
7 tbsps chia seeds**

INSTRUCTIONS

1. Add the dates, vanilla extract and the dates in a blender and blend. Resume blending on low and gradually increase to high speed till the mixture seems thoroughly smooth.
2. Now, add the raspberries together with their juice.
3. Just to combine, blend of low speed.
4. Use a spatula to stir in the chia seeds.
5. Add the chia pudding slowly to the prepared containers. (NOTE: You could use pint sized glass jars, fill them halfway to merely 1 cup mark, allowing for more space to top the pudding with fresh fruit)
6. To thicken the chia seed pudding, refrigerate for at least 5 hours or overnight.
7. Let refrigerated for 2-3 days.

The fusion of raspberry and dates is not only delightful, but also takes this recipe to the pinnacle of deliciousness. The chia pudding makes a perfectly healthy treat this fall.

LUNCH 1
AVOCADO EGG SALAD

NUTRITIONAL VALUE 155 Cal PROTEIN 9g FAT 12g
CARBOHYDRATES 4.5g

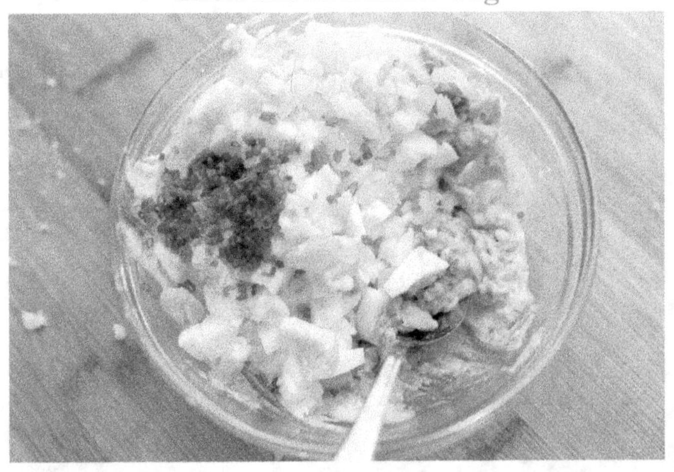

An easy to prepare, healthy to eat, and amazingly addicting avocado paleo egg salad is simply a perfect lunch idea if you were ever to throw a treat to a crowd! This recipe is perfectly Soy-free, Mayo-free, Whole30 friendly and perfectly paleo.

SERVES 4 PREPARATION TIME 5 MINUTES COOKING TIME 5 MINUTES

INGREDIENTS

5 peeled and boiled eggs

1 ripe avocado

4 slices bacon (sugar-free and nitrate-free) cooked till crumbled and crisp

2-3 finely sliced green onion

1½tbsp freshly squeezed lemon juice

½tsp sea salt, finely grained

Smoked paprika

Veggies to serve the dish with

INSTRUCTIONS

1. Chop the boiled eggs and shift them to a large bowl.
2. Cut apart the avocado and remove the pit.
3. Add the ripe avocado into the bowl.
4. Next, Mash the avocado and combine well with the freshly chopped eggs.
5. Now, add salt and the lemon juice while mixing well.
6. Add the chives, crumbled bacon and sprinkle them with the smoked paprika.
7. Serve with an extra squeeze of lemon and fresh veggies. Enjoy!

The amazing blend of avocados and eggs in a salad not only offers an absolute delight but also adds an extra-healthy parameter to this salad. So, this paleo salad makes a perfect lunch this season.

DINNER 1
ALL- HEALTHY CHICKEN PIZZA
NUTRITIONAL VALUE 135 Cal PROTEIN 6g FAT 5g
CARBOHYDRATES 15g

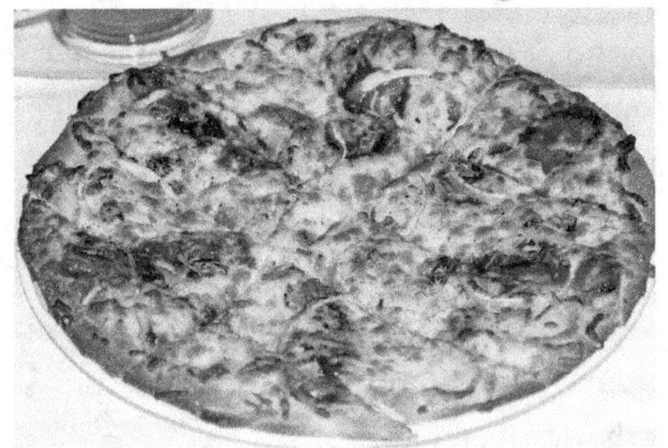

This All-Paleo chicken pizza is enriched with all the flavors of a pizza incorporated with the delicious chicken thighs. Easy, tasty, and healthy! Perfectly Paleo, Gluten free, dairy free, Whole30, it tastes incredibly amazing!

SERVES 4 PREPARATION TIME 5 MINUTES COOKING TIME 5 MINUTES

INGREDIENTS

7-8 chicken thighs

1 cup of pizza sauce (with no added sugar)

Uncured pepperoni, 24-30 slices

2 tbsp extra virgin olive oil

2 tbsp salt, for taste

1 tbsp pizza seasoning

INSTRUCTIONS

1. Preheat oven to 425degree K.
2. Add the chicken thighs to a pan: of the size 13x9.

3. Pull the skin back from each thigh and add the pizza sauce to the chicken.
4. Top each chicken thigh with 4-5 slices of pepperoni, then place the skin back over, to cover the pepperoni and sauce.
5. Lightly shower the oil on top of the chicken, drizzle with pizza seasoning and salt as per your taste.
6. Bake in the preheated oven for 40-45 minutes, or until the skin takes a brown color.

Discover the goodness of a paleo friendly pizza enriched the goodness of health and delight. Serve it with the fresh tomato ketchup and enjoy it with your loved ones.

SNACK 1
EGG MUFFIN RECIPE

NUTRITIONAL VALUE 250 Cal PROTEIN 20.3g FAT 13g
CARBOHYDRATES 6.8 g

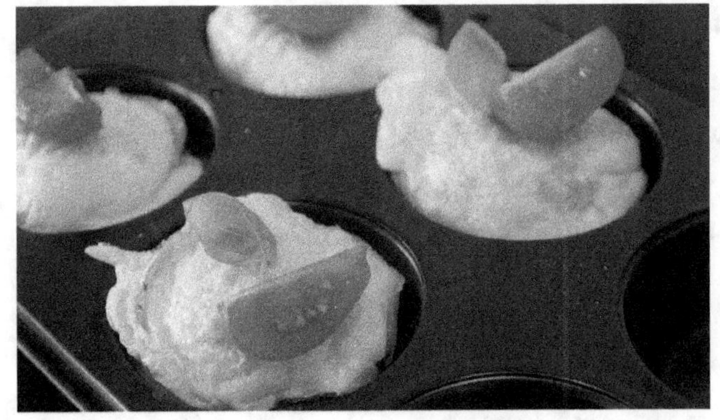

This is a Quick and Easy to prepare Paleo Egg muffin breakfast recipe that is so very convenient, enriched with flavor, veggies and meat and tastes incredibly great. Jam packed with the deliciousness, these breakfast muffins are relatively quick to be served as a breakfast.

SERVES 3 PREPARATION TIME 20MINUTES COOKING TIME 20MINUTES

INGREDIENTS

6 eggs
8 ounces crumbled and cooked ham
1 ½ cup of red bell pepper, diced
1 cup onion, diced
¼tsp salt, for taste
1 tsp ground black pepper, for taste
2 tbsp water

1. Preheat the oven to 170 degree C or 350 degrees F.
2. Drizzle 6 muffin cups and line them using a paper liner.
3. Take a large bowl and beat all the eggs within it.
4. Now, add ham, onion, bell pepper, salt, black pepper, and water into the beaten eggs.
5. Next, add the egg mixture evenly into each of the 6 muffin cups.
6. Bake the muffin cups in the preheated oven for at least 18 minutes until muffins find themselves set in the middle.

This egg muffin breakfast recipe is loaded with the goodness of a rich color, incorporated with healthy ingredient, thus making it a high protein and low carb meal.

COCONUT YOGURT PARFAIT

NUTRITIONAL VALUE 260 Cal PROTEIN 8g FAT 13g
CARBOHYDRATES 27g

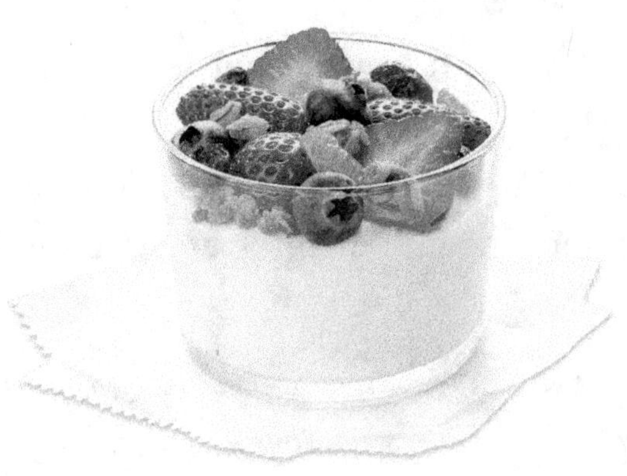

Whoever says parfait can't be paleo or healthy, haven't come across this magical coconut yogurt paleo parfait. Served aesthetically with chopped nuts, it will make you a big fan of its recipe. A quick and convenient meal ready within half an hour, this will keep your family on repeat!

SERVES 2 PREPARATION TIME 5 MINUTES
COOKING TIME 0 MINUTES

INGREDIENTS

130 ml or one pot of coconut yogurt

1 small and diced strawberry

2 raspberries

1 tsp coconut flakes
1/3 tsp cacao nibs
Chopped nuts

1. Spoon 1 tbsp of coconut yogurt into a glass or a jar. Tap the chosen utensil to make sure it comes at the bottom of the container.

2. Next, bring in the diced strawberries, coconut flakes, and the toppings of your choice. (say chopped nuts)

3. Carefully spoon another tbsp of coconut yogurt on the top of the container.

4. Place a raspberry aesthetically on the top of the parfait.

5. Serve immediately.

This Parfait has earned itself the tag of a 'crowd-pleaser' no matter where you serve it. It's not only Paleo in nature, but also assures you of its healthy features by simply being gluten-free, Whole30 and lower carb.

BREAKFAST 2
BEST BLUEBERRY CHICKEN SALAD
NUTRITIONAL VALUE 290 Cal PROTEIN 10g FAT 15g
CARBOHYDRATES 20g

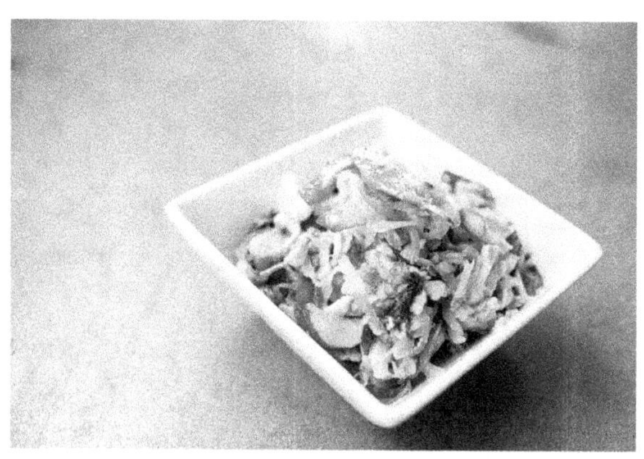

Sweet and salty – it's all in here:

Crunchy chunks of chicken elevate the delight with the addition of fresh blueberries and pleasantly odoured rosemary in this Paleo blueberry chicken salad. So let's unveil the recipe:

SERVES 4-5 PREPARATION TIME 10 MINUTES COOKING
TIME 15 MINUTES

INGREDIENTS

2 skinless, boneless chicken breasts cooked, cooled and cubed
(nearly 2 cups)

Fresh blueberries, ½ cup

Freshly Diced Celery, ¼ cup

Red onion, diced ¼ cup

3 tbsp walnuts, chopped

1 tbsp freshly chopped rosemary leaves

1/3 tsp sea salt, for taste

1/6tsp. black pepper, for taste

¼ cup mayo (Made of avocado oil)

INSTRUCTIONS

1. **How to cook chicken:** Keep a medium-large sized skillet with lid over medium-high heat.
2. Add the chicken breasts into a pan, followed by ½ cup water. Just as the water starts to boil, decrease the heat to low, cover the pan and put it on simmer for the next 15 minutes, or until the chicken is thoroughly cooked.
3. Next, place the chicken on to a plate, to let it cool before we are ready to dice.
4. **How to make salad:** Mix the cooked chicken and the left-out ingredients in a bowl.
5. Add mayo and stir gently to combine.
6. You are ready to serve the salad.

You good give this recipe a fine finishing touch by incorporating blueberries to chicken salad. This majestic recipe caters to a perfect lunch while adding a hint of splendid color, sweetness, and cancer-fighting antioxidants.

BAKED SWEET-POTATOES

NUTRITIONAL VALUE 86 Cal PROTEIN 1g FAT 3g
CARBOHYDRATES 20g

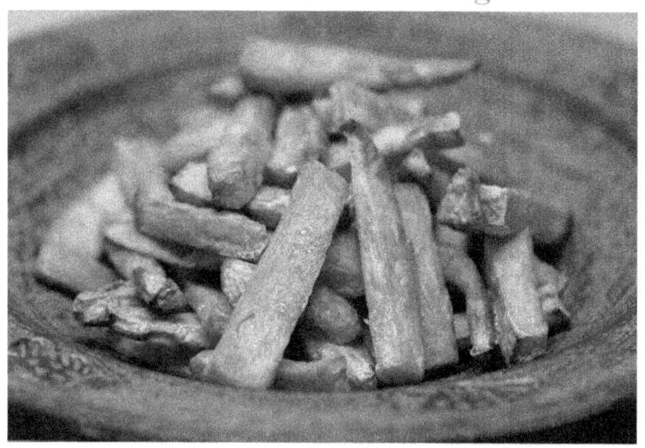

Baked Paleo sweet potatoes make a great gluten-free and paleo dinner. Be cautious in looking for small sweet potatoes that fits your fist, and be ready to cook and serve the best paleo dinner to your loved ones.

SERVES 4 PREPARATION TIME 10 MINUTES COOKING TIME 15 MINUTES

INGREDIENTS

4 sweet potatoes

1 tsp olive oil (extra-virgin)

1/3 cup water

¼ tsp kosher salt, for taste

4 tsp chives, finely chopped

INSTRUCTIONS

1. Use a fork to prick sweet potatoes and rub them with oil.
2. Add potatoes and one-quarter cup of water in a baking dish (microwave-safe); and cover with a plastic wrap.
3. Now, Microwave at high until it gets tender, for at least 15 minutes, while regularly checking for its doneness every 10 minutes. Let it cool slightly.
4. Split the potatoes partially in half lengthwise; use a fork to fluff the flesh.
5. Drizzle with salt and top thoroughly with chives.

No wonder, it's amazing to be witness to a dinner recipe steered single handed by the sweet potatoes. Furthermore, when fused with chives and salt, this recipe not only emerges delightful, but also takes health into consideration.

DINNER 2
BASIL SCRAMBLE
NUTRITIONAL VALUE 138 Cal PROTEIN 1g FAT 12g
CARBOHYDRATES 6g

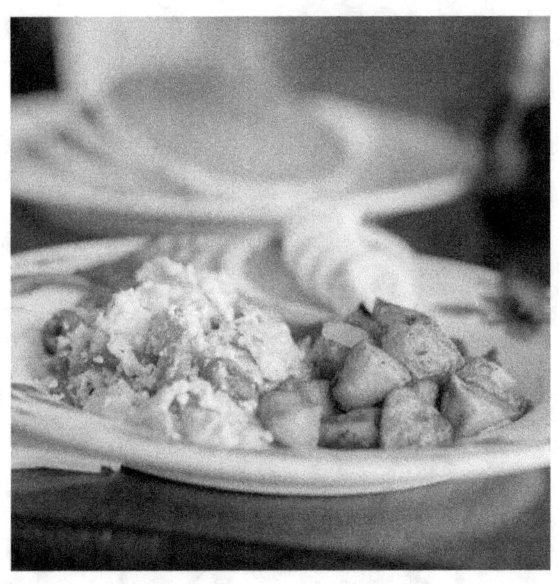

A delicious breakfast that is sure to become a prominent meal in your everyday life, the 'Gluten-free tomato basil scramble' incorporates the freshness of tomato and basil.
SERVES 4PREPARATION TIME 10MINUTES COOKING TIME 15MINUTES

INGREDIENTS
4 sweet potatoes
1 tsp olive oil (extra-virgin)
1/3 cup water
¼tsp kosher salt, for taste
4 tsp chives, finely chopped

1. Use a fork to prick sweet potatoes and rub them with oil.
2. Add potatoes and one-quarter cup of water in a baking dish (microwave-safe); and cover with a plastic wrap.
3. Now, Microwave at high until it gets tender, for at least 15 minutes, while regularly checking for its doneness every 10 minutes. Let it cool slightly.
4. Split the potatoes partially in half lengthwise; use a fork to fluff the flesh.
5. Drizzle with salt and top thoroughly with chives.

The gluten free tomato basil scramble recipe simply turns simple scrambled eggs into a marvelous treat. It ensures you a full and satisfied meal, no matter what. Enjoy!

EASY GAZPACHO

NUTRITIONAL VALUE 130 Cal PROTEIN 2g FAT 6g
CARBOHYDRATES 17g

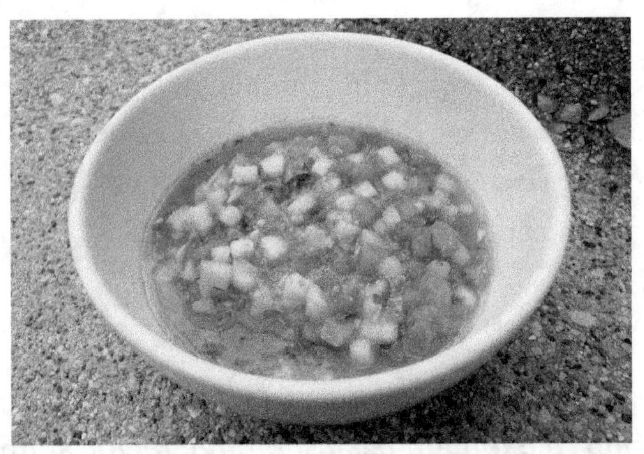

A naturally paleo and gluten-free blend of nearly the maximum number of vegetables one could fit into one bowl, Gazpacho is your one-stop recipe that's refreshing and makes for a health-studded lunch.

SERVES 4-6PREPARATION TIME 10MINUTES COOKING TIME 0MINUTES

INGREDIENTS

Cucumber, slashed into half

1 red and green pepper each

4 tomatoes, vined

1 medium-large sized onion

1 hot pepper

1 small-cup of tomato juice

1 cup vinegar (red wine)

½ tsp salt and freshly ground pepper, for taste

INSTRUCTIONS

1. Take a blender and add half of the cucumber, pepper and onion to it and blend till the vegetables are finely chopped.
2. Remove the apparatus from the blender and keep it aside.
3. Next, add the remaining cucumber, onion and peppers to the blender and blend the apparatus till it is finely chopped. Now, bring in the tomato juice and keep blending till the mixture becomes smooth.
4. Add the red wine vinegar, ground pepper and sea salt and blend until the mixture is combined well.
5. Add tomato mixture to the **veggies chopped in the first step,** and stir well to form a thick soup.
6. Place the soup in an airtight container and refrigerate for at least 3 hours to allow the flavors to meld.
7. You can continue to enjoy it while keeping it in refrigerator for up to 1 week.

Loaded with the goodness of the refreshing cucumber, this paleo gazpacho naturally balances the tartness of tomatoes and the sweetness of bell peppers, making it an absolute lunch delight.

DESSERT 2
COCNUT TRUFFLES
NUTRITIONAL VALUE 230 Cal PROTEIN 2g FAT 18g
CARBOHYDRATES 16g

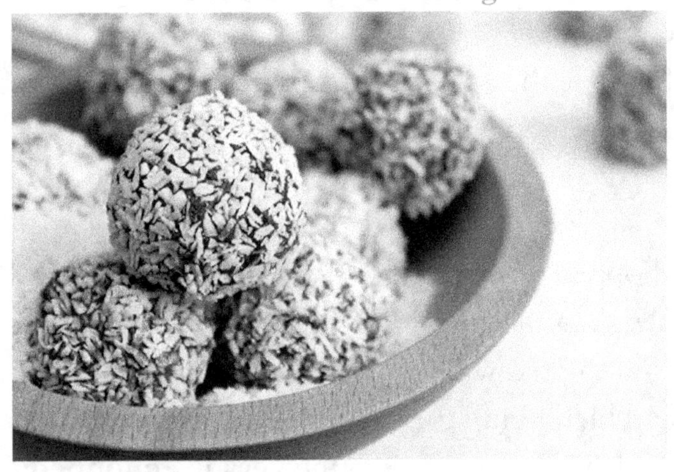

INGREDIENTS

2 boxes of confectioners' sugar-free sugar (16 ounces)

1 (14 ounce) can of sweetened milk

1 cup of butter

2 ½ cups of walnuts, chopped

1 package of coconut (14 ounce and shredded)

1 bag of chocolate chips (24 ounces)

INSTRUCTIONS

1. Use a waxed paper to line the baking sheet.

2. Next, mix the (sugar-free) sugar, sweetened condensed milk, and butter together in a bowl.

3. Stir the coconuts and walnuts into dough.

4. Carefully cover the bowl using a plastic wrap and let the dough freeze until it grows firm for at least 1 hour.

5. Carefully make 1-inch balls using the dough, and place these balls on the prepared baking sheet, and let it freeze for at least 30 minutes.

6. Let the coconut melt in a double boiler filled with simmering water while stirring frequently or until it gets smooth.

7. Last but not the least, plunge balls within the melted chocolate and coat it nicely; allow it to cool on prepared baking sheet till chocolate gets hard enough.

This makes a great recipe for the coming holidays! Get set to give it all to your friends and family at Christmas time. But remember: Do not allow the balls sit in the chocolate for long or they might just melt.

EGG CASSEROLES

NUTRITIONAL VALUE 334 Cal PROTEIN 17g FAT 23g
CARBOHYDRATES 14g

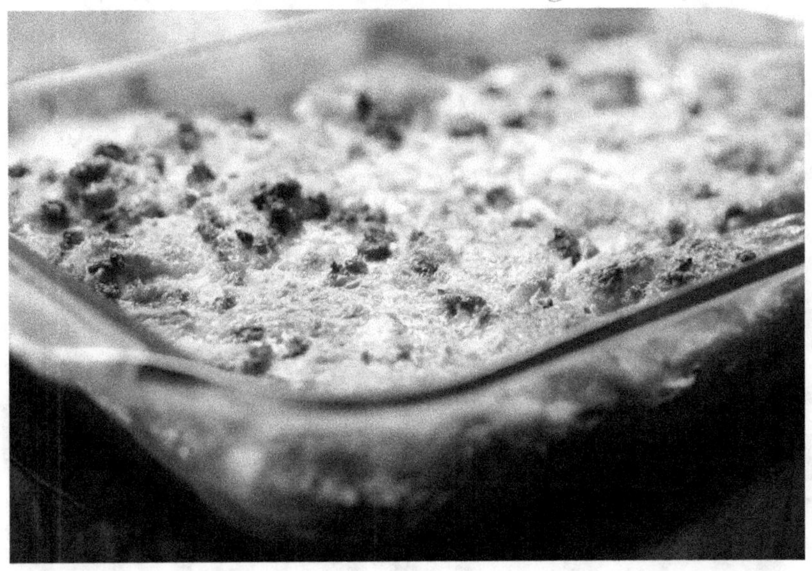

An easy to prepare, healthy to eat, and amazingly addicting Paleo Egg Casseroles are simply a perfect breakfast idea if you were ever to throw a treat to a crowd! This recipe is perfectly Soy-free, Mayo-free, Whole30 friendly and perfectly paleo.

SERVES 4PREPARATION TIME 10MINUTES COOKING TIME 10MINUTES

INGREDIENTS

Paleo Breakfast Sausage, ½lb

Diced Broccoli, ½ cup

½ diced Onion

6Eggs

1 diced tomato
1 diced bell pepper
Sea Salt and black pepper to taste

INSTRUCTIONS
1. Preheat the oven to 350 degrees F.
2. Add the eggs in a medium sized bowl and beat them until they start frothing.
3. Bring the onion, sausage, pepper, broccoli and tomato and stir well to combine these ingredients.
4. Distribute the mixture evenly among 6 different serving dishes.
5. Season with the sea salt and pepper.
6. Cook the mixture in the preheated oven for nearly 10 minutes, or till the eggs become firm.
7. Serve immediately.

The rich fusion of sausage, broccoli and onions make this recipe a true Morning delight. Besides taking you to the pinnacle of deliciousness, this recipe makes a perfectly healthy treat this fall.

LUNCH 3
POMEGRANATE CURRY CHICKEN

NUTRITIONAL VALUE 238 Cal PROTEIN 29g FAT 11g
CARBOHYDRATES 3g

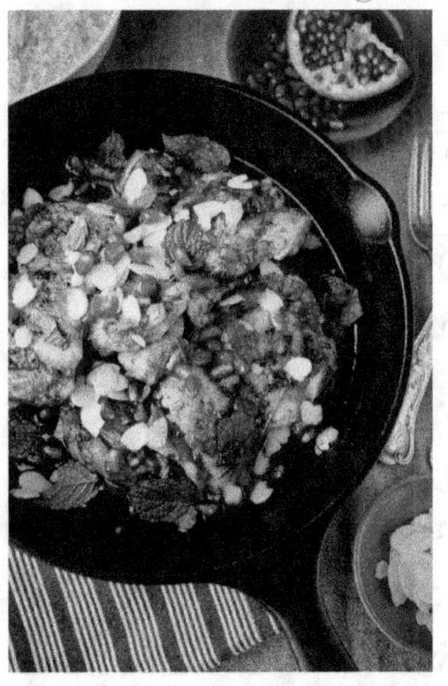

No matter if you serve this easy and elegant pomegranate curry chicken with a bed of greens or with a side of steamed broccoli, it will quickly become your favorite recipe for dinner.

SERVES 4 PREPARATION TIME 10 MINUTES COOKING TIME 10 MINUTES

INGREDIENTS

3-oz. of boneless, skinless chicken thighs

1 tsp curry powder

½tsp kosher salt

½tsp black pepper for taste

1½ tsp olive oil (extra-virgin)

¼ cup pomegranate arils

2 tsp mint leaves, torn

1. Drizzle the whole of the chicken with salt, pepper and curry powder.
2. Pre-heat the oil over medium to high heat in a large-size skillet.
3. Add the chicken to this skillet and cook for the next 5 minutes on both the sides or until completely done.
4. Next, shift the chicken to the serving-platter.
5. You are ready to serve the chicken, just drizzle it with mint and pomegranate arils and enjoy a quick meal.

This chicken dish makes a perfect dinner, as it requires handful of preparation and is ready to serve almost immediately. So get set for this dreamy dinner and enjoy!

DINNER 3
GRILLED FISH FILLET

NUTRITIONAL VALUE 123 Cal PROTEIN 25.53g FAT 1.33g
CARBOHYDRATES 0.31g

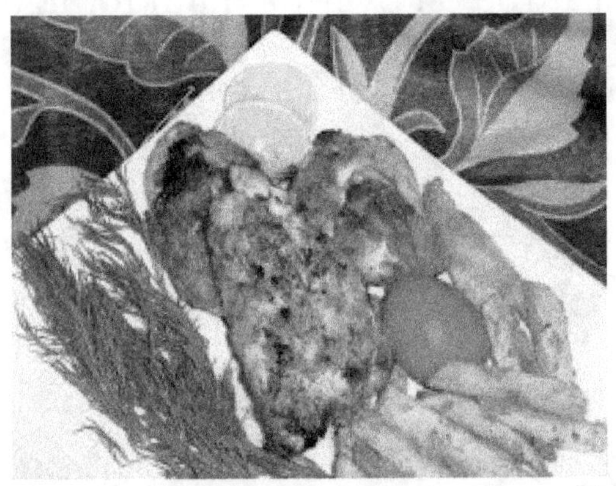

This dinner couldn't have met a simpler fate. Made from the wholesome and delicious ingredients, these gluten-free grilled fish skillet is best served fresh, so prepare the skillet and gift yourself the luxury of a delicious fish skillet.
SERVES 4PREPARATION TIME 10MINUTES COOKING TIME 15MINUTES

INGREDIENTS

4 (5 oz) of porgy fillets
4 teaspoons of olive oil
Salt and freshly ground pepper, to taste
4 fresh sprig herbs (rosemary, parsley, oregano)
1 thinly sliced lemon
4 large pieces (20 inch) of heavy duty aluminum foil

INSTRUCTIONS

1. Line the fish at the center of the foil.
2. Season with salt and pepper as per your taste while drizzling with olive oil.
3. Add a slice of lemon on the top of each fish piece, followed by a sprig of herbs on each.
4. Deliberately fold up the edges, to make surethat it's thoroughly sealed and no steam escaped.
5. Be careful in heating just one half of the grill on high heat while closing off the cover.
6. And when the grill is adequately hot, keep the foil packets beside the grill while the burner is turned off.
7. You can cook according to the thickness of your fish, for 10 to 15 minutes, or until it is adequately cooked through.

The fusion of fillets and herbs is not only taste-full, but also takes this recipe to the pinnacle of deliciousness. So, the fish skillet makes a perfectly healthy treat this fall.

ALMOND BUTTER-BANANA COOKIES

NUTRITIONAL VALUE 62.7 Cal PROTEIN 1.3g FAT 2g
CARBOHYDRATES 10.5g

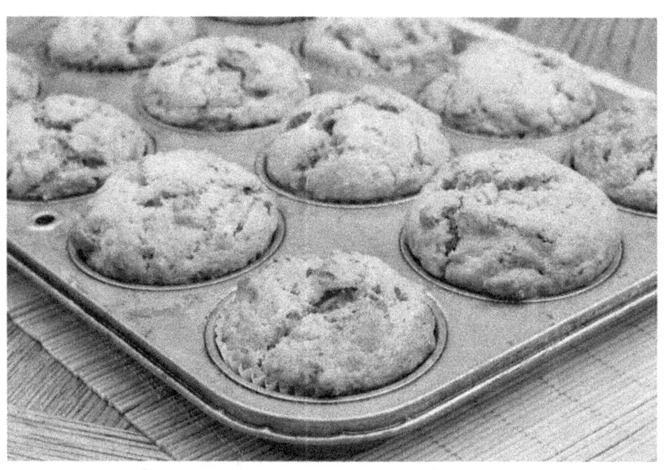

*This breakfast recipe couldn't have met a simpler fate.
Made from the wholesome and delicious ingredients,
these paleo cookies are best eaten fresh, so prepare the
batter and have the leverage to make whenever you want
to eat them.*

SERVES 14PREPARATION TIME 40MINUTES COOKING
TIME 40MINUTES

INGREDIENTS

1Egg

Maple syrup, 3tbsp

Vanilla extract, 2tsp

Almond butter, 1cup

1Ripe Banana

INSTRUCTIONS

1. Bring all the ingredients together in a food processor. Blend thoroughly well it becomes a smooth mixture.
2. Keep this batter into the refrigerator for at least 30 minutes, all allow it to cool.
3. Keep your oven ready by preheating it at 325 degree K and line a baking sheet with parchment paper.
4. Add the batter to the required number of cookies onto the baking sheet, whereas setting aside the remaining batter for the next batch. Stay assured, the batter could endure up to 3 days in the refrigerator.
5. Allow the batter-stuffed cookies to be baked in the preheated oven for at least 10 minutes, or until these cookies turn brownish on the bottom.
6. Place these cookies on a cooling rack for atleast 5 minutes.
7. Serve warm.

There are no second opinions that the banana paleo cookies are driven by the goodness of banana and vanilla extracts. Furthermore, when fused almond butter and maple syrup, this recipe not only emerges delightful, but also takes health into consideration.

DESSERT 3

SWEET BARS

NUTRITIONAL VALUE 75 Cal PROTEIN 5.3g FAT 1.6g
CARBOHYDRATES 6.5g

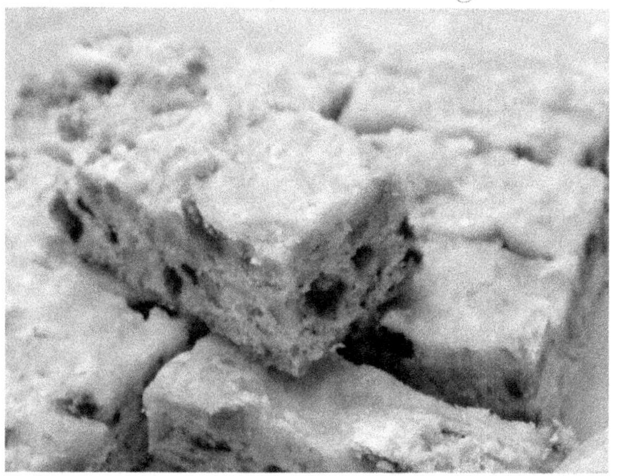

These PALEO BARS make it way easier to get through your day by bidding an adieu to hunger no matter when. A fact that will make you feel good about these bars is they are absolutely paleo-friendly and carefully designed to cater to you the clean burning energy with no crash later.

INGREDIENTS

2 medium-sized cups of your favorite mixed nuts

1 cup of dates

1/3 cup of cacao powder

2 tbsp coconut oil

INSTRUCTIONS

1. Process your favourite nuts in a food processor. until very fine.

2. Add the cacao powder and coconut oil to the food processor and process it until it creates fudgy and sticky dough.
3. Line a square sized pan with a baking paper.
4. Carefully spread the mixture into the pan and keep into the fridge to set.
5. When you are all set, cut the bars into small pieces and enjoy.
6. Store in the fridge.

What sets these bars apart and make them more beautiful is the addition of dates and chocolate that not only enhance their taste but also make it extra satisfying because of the nuts they contain.

BREAKFAST 4
BLACKENED STEAK SALAD

NUTRITIONAL VALUE 332 Cal PROTEIN 21g FAT 24.4g
CARBOHYDRATES 6g

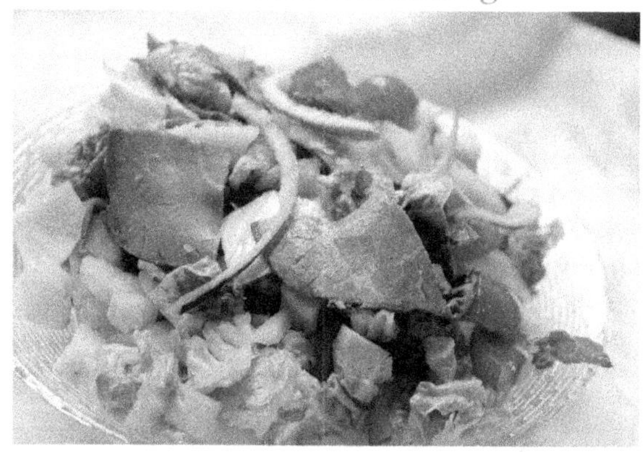

Steak-centric salads often feature in the English gastro pub menu. Catering the royal menu to your doorsteps: this salad incorporates char grilled steak, topped with avocado and a vinaigrette that elevates the veggies rather than disguise them. This recipe is not only healthy but also paleo-friendly.

SERVES 4PREPARATION TIME 15MINUTES COOKING TIME 10MINUTES

INGREDIENTS

½ tsp kosher salt

½ tsp black pepper

½ tsp paprika

¼ tsp garlic powder

12 oz. of trimmed flank steak

¼ cups of olive oil (extra-virgin)

2 tbsp balsamic vinegar

1 tsp Dijon mustard
4 cups arugula, firmly packed
½ red onion, vertically sliced
½ chopped ripe avocado

INSTRUCTIONS

1. Take a grill pan and heat it over the medium to high heat.
2. In a small bowl add salt, pepper and garlic powder; mix it all thoroughly.
3. Rub the spice mixture thoroughly and evenly over the steak. Bring the steak into pan; let it grill for at least 5 minutes on both the sides until you reach the desired degree of doneness.
4. Keep the steak on to a cutting board. Let it cool for 5 minutes. Now, cut the grain into thin slices.
5. Next, mix vinegar, oil and mustard in a large bowl, while regularly stirring with a whisk.
6. Add arugula, steak and onion; toss to coat.
7. Divide salad among 4 plates and dress evenly with avocado.

This is a Quick and Easy to prepare breakfast salad recipe that is so very convenient, enriched with flavor, and tastes incredibly great. Enriched with the deliciousness, this breakfast salad is relatively quick to be served as a breakfast.

GOOD AFTERNOON PIZZA SOUP

NUTRITIONAL VALUE 224.7 Cal PROTEIN 6.9g FAT 16.4g
CARBOHYDRATES 8.3g

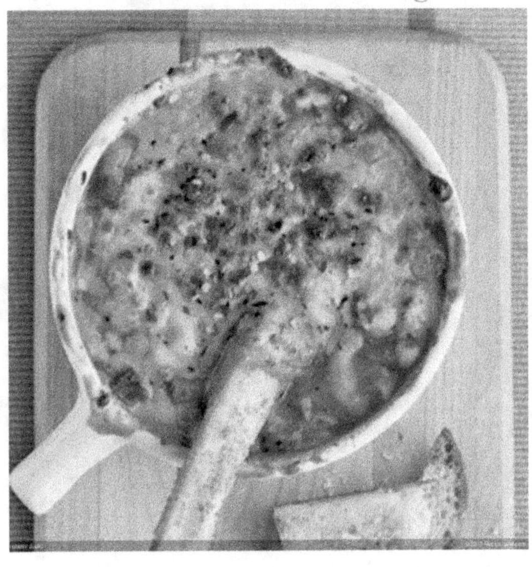

What makes this Good Afternoon pizza soup a delicious lunch recipe is the fact that it could be customized as per your needs. Don't like peppers? Leave them out. Love mushrooms? Add them. So, no matter what you like, simply add it on the pizza. To keep is healthy and clean we used a chicken sausage that is absolutely Whole30 in nature, but you are free to use both ground sausage and ground beef.

SERVES 4 PREPARATION TIME 15MINUTES COOKING TIME 10MINUTES

INGREDIENTS

12 oz of sliced and diced chicken sausage

4 oz of uncured pepperoni, chopped into 4ths
1 jar of marinara (25 oz)
1 can of the fire roasted tomatoes (14.5 oz)
1 medium-large diced onion
16oz of sliced mushrooms
1 can of sliced black olives (3oz)
1 tbsp of the dried oreganos
1 tsp garlic powder
½ tsp salt, for taste

INSTRUCTIONS

1. Combine pepperoni, marinara, onion, tomatoes, mushrooms, olives, oregano and garlic powder, in a large sized bowl.
2. Take a large sized saucepan to mix well the sausage and pepperoni.
3. Cook the mixture over medium to high heat for nearly half an hour or until mushrooms and onions have softened.
4. Add salt as per your taste.
5. Serve hot and makes great leftovers.

This good afternoon lunch recipe is an absolute crowd pleaser, no matter if you serve it on an occasion or to your special one. Besides being paleo in nature, it also assures of its health benefits by simply being gluten-free, Whole30 and lower carb.

PUMPKIN CHILI

NUTRITIONAL VALUE 409 Cal PROTEIN 28.4g FAT 16.4g
CARBOHYDRATES 37.3g

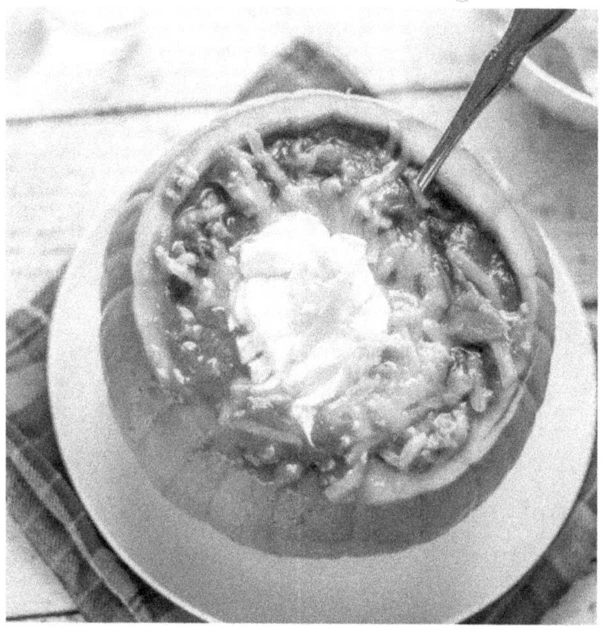

This dinner recipe couldn't have met a simpler and more convenient fate. Made from the wholesome and delicious ingredients, this paleo pumpkin chili is best eaten fresh, so get set for this health-studded paradise.

SERVES 4 PREPARATION TIME 15 MINUTES COOKING TIME
30 MINUTES

INGREDIENTS

3 cups of yellow onion, chopped
7 garlic cloves, chopped

Ground turkey, 1 pound
2 cans (15 oz each) of fire-roasted tomatoes
1 ½ cups of pumpkin puree
1 cup of chicken broth
2 tbsp of honey
4 tsp of dried oregano
2 tsp of chili spice
1 tsp of ground cinnamon
1 tsp of sea salt for taste

INSTRUCTIONS

1. Saute' the garlic and the onions in coconut oil for nearly five to six minutes.
2. Bring in the ground turkey and try breaking it up using a spatula and allow it to cook for the next five minutes.
3. Slowly add the remaining ingredients while stirring the and gradually bringing them to a simmer.
4. Allow it to simmer without the help of a lid for the next 15 minutes.
5. You can introduce more and more chicken broth to add thinness if desired.
6. Finally, you can serve with a big salad.

Additional tip: You can prepare this beanless chili on a Sunday. Enriched with the goodness of protein and extra hearty cups of pumpkin puree, it'll take away the thinking out of dinner during your hectic work routine.

BUTTER SCALLOPS

NUTRITIONAL VALUE 215.6 Cal PROTEIN 38.7g FAT 13.8g
CARBOHYDRATES 11.0g

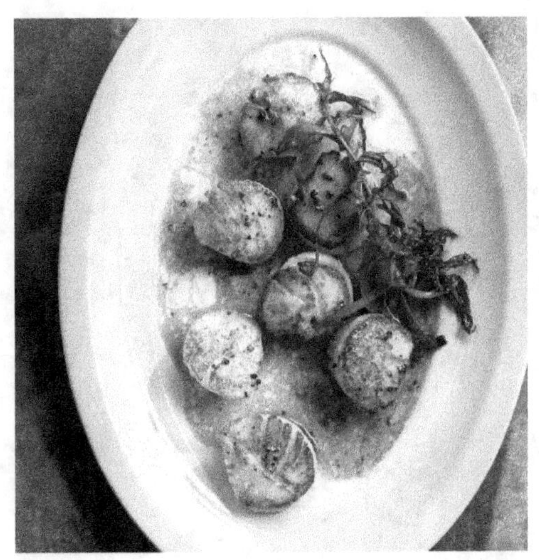

If you are fond of the butter chicken, then you can get the
same sort of taste only with these Paleo Butter Scallops
recipe. Don't be scared of the long-list of the ingredients. All
it takes is one pan to combine everything as instructed in the
tutorial and you are ready with your breakfast within 25
minutes.

SERVES 3-4 PREPARATION TIME 10 MINUTES COOKING
TIME 15 MINUTES

INGREDIENTS

2 tbsp ghee
1 cup of the minced shallot
2 tsp garlic paste (fresh)
2 tsp of fresh ginger paste

¼ cup of fresh tomato paste
½ tsp of salt for taste
1 tsp garam masala
Pinch of cayenne pepper
¼ tsp of ground cumin
¼ tsp of ground cinnamon
½ pound of sea scallops
8 ounces of cream' fraiche
Fresh cilantro for garnishing purpose

INSTRUCTIONS

1. Heat the ghee over medium-high heat in a large skillet or wok pan.
2. Introduce the shallot and cook, while stirring gently and frequently, till the ingredient starts to get tender.
3. Bring in the ginger paste, garlic paste, tomato paste, garam masala, salt, cayenne, cumin, and cinnamon, and proceed towards cooking for the next 5 minutes.
4. Add the scallops and creme fraiche, continue cooking until the scallops are thoroughly cooked through.
5. Garnish with the fresh cilantro and serve.

Ready to serve within 25 minutes from the start, the dish will cherish your name amongst your guests or it works wonders as just as a treat to yourself. And, last but not the least, it is Paleo-approved.

DESSERT 4
BANANA AND BACON

NUTRITIONAL VALUE 75 Cal PROTEIN 5.3g FAT 1.6g
CARBOHYDRATES 6.5g

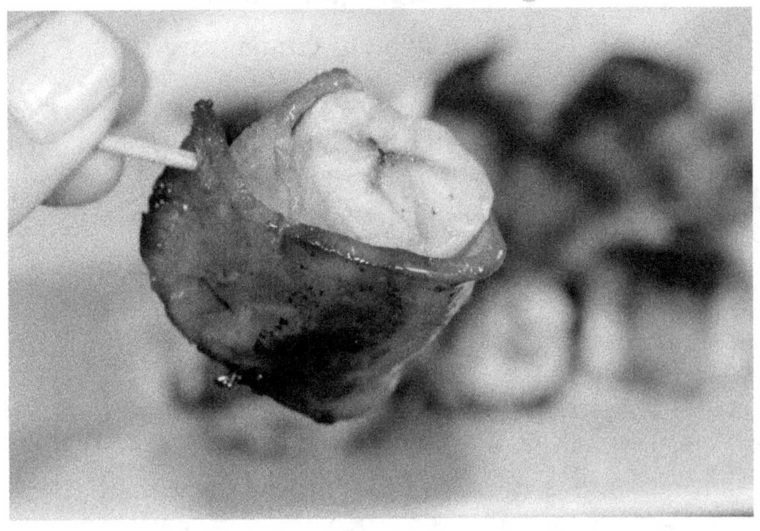

This dessert might seems strange at first, but we are sure this sweet and innovative recipe will become a prominent recipe in your dessert menu.

SERVES 3 PREPARATION TIME 5 MINUTES
COOKING TIME 5 MINUTES

INGREDIENTS

3 chopped pieces of bacon
1 sliced banana
Optional Maple syrup for drizzling on top

1. Chop the pieces of bacon in a pan and let them fry over the medium-high heat.
2. Bring in the sliced banana as soon as you realize the bacon turns brown and formed grease in the pan.
3. Turn over the banana pieces to let them turn brown on both the sides.
4. At last, spray the recipe with the maple syrup and you are ready to serve.

Bacons are not generally known for quick, simple and cheap meal, but with this paleo recipe you will realize it's a big mistake. They are pretty inexpensive workable and they get ready to be served in a really quick time. Also a great occasion food, it's something you are actually missing on your paleo diet.

PANCETTA AND FIGS

NUTRITIONAL VALUE 190 Cal PROTEIN 3.4g FAT 3g
CARBOHYDRATES 28g

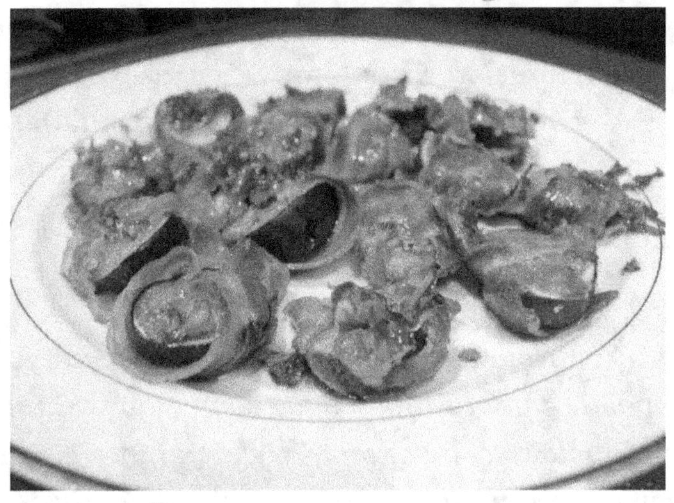

If you like to try new and healthy things, then you would love the combination of figs and pancetta. What lies in between the pancetta and figs are basil leaves, so you are assured of the tons of flavor from merely a few simple ingredients.

SERVES 3-4 PREPARATION TIME 10 MINUTES COOKING TIME 20 MINUTES

INGREDIENTS

5 black figs
10 basil leaves, fresh
10 slices prosciutto or pancetta
Olive oil

Toothpicks

Balsamic vinegar

INSTRUCTIONS

1. Heat the oven in advance at 375 degree K.

2. Line a baking sheet together with a foil.

3. You can gently brush the foil using a little olive oil. Moreover, you could chop the figs in half after taking the stems off.

4. Keep a basil leaf right on the cut side of each fig half, followed by wrapping it with a piece of pancetta and finally securing with a toothpick.

5. Bake the ingredient for the next 20 minutes, while rotating the pan once. The pancetta must have turned little bit browned and sizzling by now.

6. Serve hot or warm, and sprinkle with a little balsamic vinegar.

This lunch recipe is as easy and convenient as tooth-picking some pancetta and figs and baking them up. And if you serve them up as appetizers, your party comers will simply think you're the next celebrity chef.

INDIAN RAINBOW SALAD

NUTRITIONAL VALUE 225 Cal PROTEIN 12g FAT 0g
CARBOHYDRATES 14g

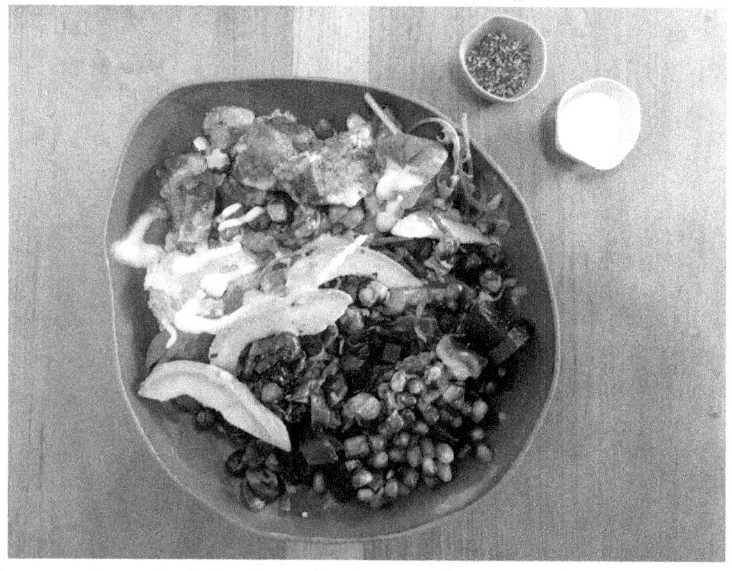

This veggie-salad derives its roots from India and has a lot
going on, but is still way, way easy and convenient to make.
Soon to be your favorite breakfast to turn to, the Indian
rainbow salad comes loaded with the goodness of the healthy
veggie you need to sustain a paleo-friendly diet.

INGREDIENTS

For the salad:

Arugula
1 or 2 carrots
½ head of red cabbage
½ mangos
Handful of cilantro

2 ½ green onion stalk
Handful of cashews

For the dressing:

1/3 cups of lime juice
2 tbsp brown sugar
3 tbsp fish sauce
Optional red pepper flakes

INSTRUCTIONS

For the salad:
1. Cut the carrots, mango and red cabbage into finer slices.
2. Chop the green onions and cilantro.
3. Next, allow the cashews to be toasted.
4. Toss the chopped vegetables in step 1, fruits and arugula with the chopped cilantro and green onions.

For the dressing:

1. Add the brown sugar, lime juice, fish sauce and red pepper flakes in a jar and shake the mixture to dissolve the sugar.
2. Toss the salad with the dressing.

The amazing blend of veggies and fruits in the Indian rainbow salad not only offers an absolute delight but also adds an extra-healthy parameter to this salad. So, this paleo salad makes a perfect breakfast this season.

DINNER 5
CHICKEN TERIYAKI

NUTRITIONAL VALUE 342 Cal PROTEIN 52g FAT 7g
CARBOHYDRATES 12g

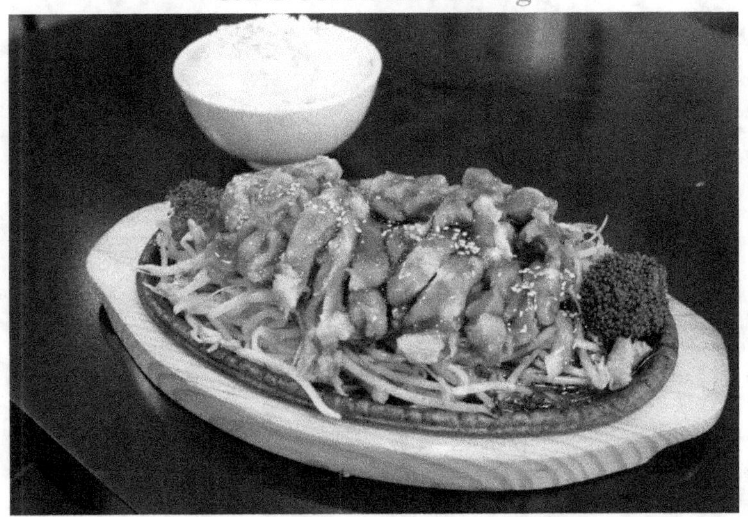

The fusion of chicken and teriyaki sauce is not only taste-full, but also takes this recipe to the pinnacle of deliciousness. So, the Paleo Chicken Teriyaki makes a perfectly healthy treat this fall.

SERVES 2 PREPARATION TIME 10 MINUTES COOKING TIME 20 MINUTES

INGREDIENTS

1 ½ lbs chicken thigh skin on-2 pieces

Salt to taste

½ tbsp ghee / oil to pan fry the chicken

Toasted white sesame seeds (optional)

TERIYAKI SAUCE

2 ½ tbsp coconut aminos

1 tbsp ginger garlic paste
1 tbsp apple cider vinegar
¾ tbsp red boat fish sauce

INSTRUCTIONS

1. Heat 1/2 tbsp ghee over medium/high heat. When hot, add chicken and pan fry about 10 minutes until both sides of the chicken get crispy.
2. Drain the extra oil and keep the chicken aside.
3. **Make the sauce:** In the same sauce pan, add all the ingredients of the teriyaki sauce mentioned above and heat the pan over medium heat.
4. When the sauce is thickened, add the chicken to it . Coat the saucer over the chicken well.
5. Add white sesame seeds and let the chicken absorb the sauce.

For Garnish-

Wait for 5 minutes before serving, when cooled down serve with rice.

This makes a great recipe for the coming holidays! Get set to give it all to your friends and family at Christmas time. But remember: Do not allow the balls sit in the chocolate for long or they might just melt.

BANANA COCONUT AND MILK ICE-CREAM

NUTRITIONAL VALUE 190 Cal PROTEIN 12g FAT 4.5 g
CARBOHYDRATES 14 g

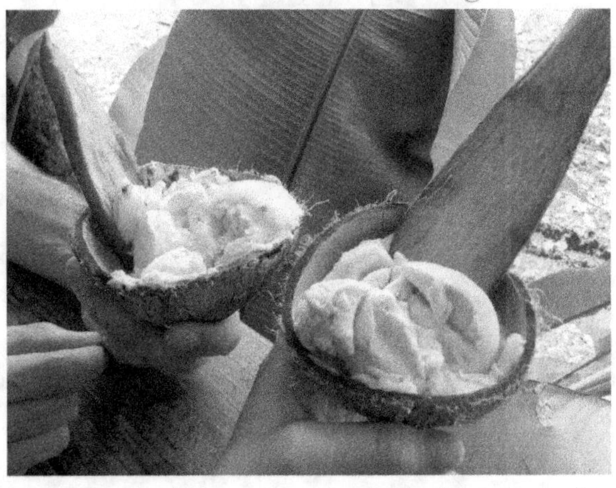

Who says there are no ice-creams included in the paleo diet? This ice-cream is one of the best ways to keep yourself updated with the desserts and remind yourself that dieting doesn't have to be a chore or a sacrifice.

SERVES 3-4 PREPARATION TIME 2 Hours COOKING TIME 15 MINUTES

INGREDIENTS

1 tbsp melted coconut oil
3 medium peeled and sliced bananas
1 can of coconut milk (full fat)

INSTRUCTIONS

1. Preheat your oven to 400 degree K.

2. Add the banana slice to the rimmed baking dish and sprinkle with coconut oil.
3. Bake the banana slice for the next 20 minutes, unless and until it gets tender, while tossing in between.
4. Shift the cooked banana slices to a blender while scraping your pan to incorporate the syrup cooked out from the bananas.
5. Add coconut milk and blend until they are combined smoothly.
6. Chill the mixture for 4 hours minimum.
7. Freeze in accordance with the ice cream maker's instructions.
8. Store in an airtight freezer-safe container for 1 week.

This recipe is perfectly illustrates that you do not require a cow to enjoy ice cream, as it is made of coconut milk, it will be rich and creamy with a slight coconut flavor.

DESSERT 5
APPLE PIE

NUTRITIONAL VALUE 230 Cal PROTEIN 2g FAT 8 g
CARBOHYDRATES 37 g

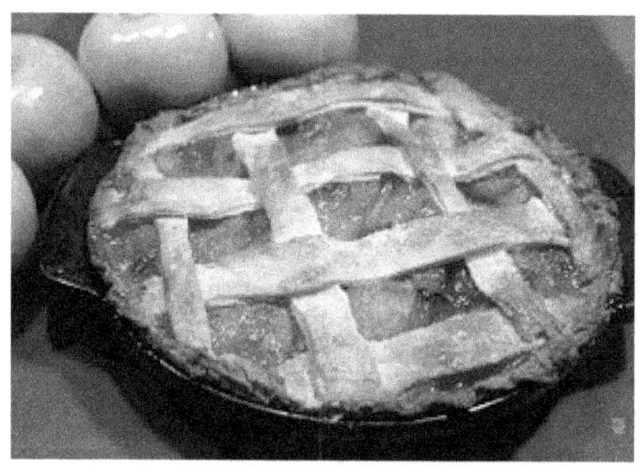

INGREDIENTS

1. **6** cups thinly sliced, peeled apples (6 medium)

2. **¾** cup sugar

3. **2** tsp all-purpose flour

4. **¾** teaspoon ground cinnamon

5. **¼** teaspoon salt

6. **1** tsp ground nutmeg

7. **1** tsp lemon juice

Nutritional information: 230 calories per serving.

INSTRUCTIONS

1. Preheat oven to 425°F. Add 1 pie crust in 9-inch glass pie plate.

2. Add filling ingredients to a large bowl, mix gently; add spoon by spoon into pie plate lined with crust. Next, top with second crust. Cut shapes or slits in numerous places in top crust.

3. Next, bake for 45 minutes or until apples turn soft and tender. Prevent excess browning by covering edge of crust with 2-inch wide foil strips. Allow it to cool on the cooling rack for 1 hour before serving.

BREAKFAST 6
CHIPS AND FISH

NUTRITIONAL VALUE 310 Cal PROTEIN 27g FAT 18.4 g
CARBOHYDRATES 36 g

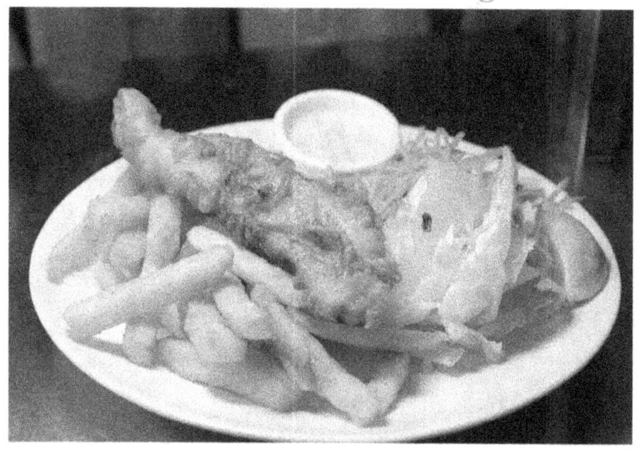

No matter fish and chips is the classic British version of fast food, the recipe perfectly falls under the guidelines of a paleo diet. The fish gets the luxury of being coated in almond flour whereas the chips derive their base material from the sweet potatoes. Fried in the Paleo-friendly oil, they could make you fall for their classic deep fried taste.

SERVES 3 PREPARATION TIME 5 MINUTES COOKING TIME
10 MINUTES

INGREDIENTS

1 lb of cod (wild and caught)
2 ½ cups of paleo-friendly coconut oil for frying
1 ½ cup of almond flour
2 eggs
½ cup of coconut milk
1 tsp. sea salt

INSTRUCTIONS

1. Combine the eggs, sea salt, almond flour, and coconut milk in a blender or food processor.
2. Mix well.
3. Carefully chop the cod into fine strips.
4. Heat the paleo-friendly coconut oil on the stove.
5. Batter the cod and continue frying until it turns golden brown in color.
6. Enjoy!

This recipe is delicious enough to tantalize your taste buds. In fact you will be amazed that you could throw it together in no time at all. Provided it's super easy to make so you can make a batch of it and use it for serving your guests no matter when.

SALMON SALAD

NUTRITIONAL VALUE 200 Cal PROTEIN 11g FAT 20g
CARBOHYDRATES 1 g

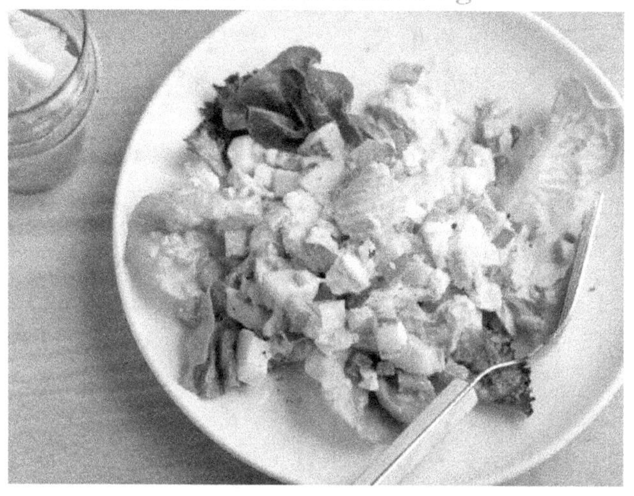

This is one such insanely easily made dish, perfect for lunch on the go and also rich in protein and a good source of omega-3 fatty acids. Salmon Salad is a 5 minute cook.

SERVES 4 PREPARATION TIME 5 MINUTES COOKING TIME
5 MINUTES

INGREDIENTS

10-12 oz. canned mayonnaise

4 tbsp celery chopped

2 tbsp of chopped onion

1/2 tsp. Dried dill

A pinch of black pepper

1. Take a bowl and add the all the ingredients and toss them properly.
2. Take a kale leaf or collard, on a bed of greens, add veggies such as cucumber, tomato on the top and roll over.

Life is busy, but don't let that disrupt your lifestyle in any way, choose this healthy option!

DINNER 6
TOMATO AND BASIL CHICKEN

NUTRITIONAL VALUE 220 Cal PROTEIN 30g FAT 10g
CARBOHYDRATES 4 g

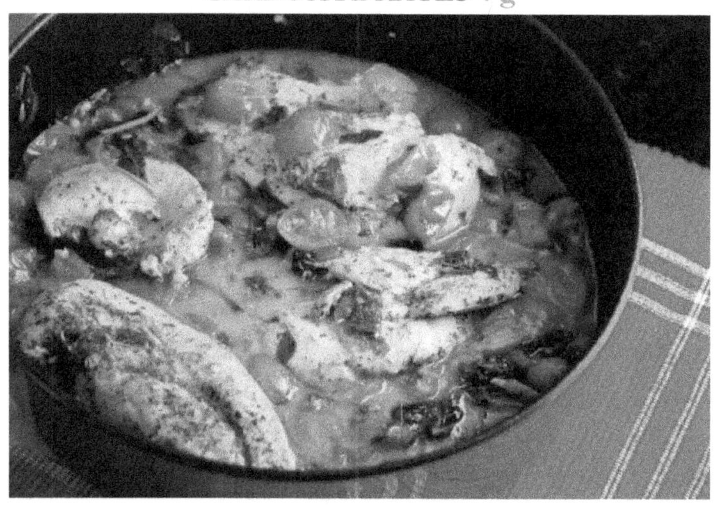

Paleo diets focus on grass-fed meats a lot, chicken is a great option for dinner. Give a tangy hint to your chicken, how about chicken tossed in pesto!

SERVES 2 PREPARATION TIME 15 MINUTES COOKING TIME
30 MINUTES

INGREDIENTS

2 pound chicken thighs/breasts, boneless and skinless

1 onion, yellow

2 teaspoon coconut oil

1 teaspoon arrowroot powder

½ cup cold water

1 cup coconut milk

Nut-Free Dairy-Free Pesto:

5 cloves of garlic

4 tbsp. sunflower seeds

2 ½ tbsp. nutritional yeast

Handful of salt & pepper

1 (2-3) oz. package fresh basil

2 tbsp. avocado oil

INSTRUCTIONS

1. In a medium-sized skillet, heat coconut oil over medium-high or until it starts to sizzle.
2. Meanwhile, chop the onion into strips; add to the pan; cook until it becomes translucent.
3. Next, add chicken; cook for another 15 minutes; flip over; cook for 15 more minutes or until there's no pink in the middle of the chicken.

Prepare the pesto:

1. Add garlic in a food processor; Pulse until finely minced. Next, add sunflower seeds, pulse.

2. Add nutrition yeast, salt, a dash of pepper to the food processor. Lastly, add avocado oil and basil.

3. Pulse until the basil is well minced. Meanwhile, as you prepare the recipe, you could set the pesto aside.

4. In a bowl, add arrowroot powder and water and whisk them together.

5. Add the coconut milk, and then whisk in the pesto.

6. Add the sauce to the chicken resting within the skillet and bring it to simmer.

7. Add the sliced cherry tomatoes and let it simmer for another couple of minutes or until tomatoes become warm. Serve.

This cuisine is a creamy yet tangy, you can serve this with zoodles as an optional method but it serves quite a meal itself

SNACK 6
BANANA AVOCADO BLUEBERRY TRIO
NUTRITIONAL VALUE 124Cal PROTEIN 5g FAT 6.8 g
CARBOHYDRATES 14g

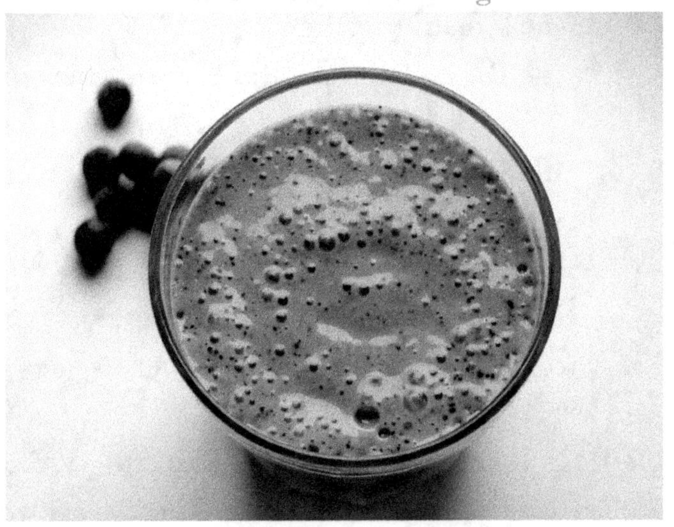

In Paleo diet fresh fruits play a very essential part. Go for the seasonal fruits and make their shakes and smoothies for breakfast options. Natural fructose provides a superb taste also adds nuts to complete the meal.

SERVES 1 PREPARATION TIME 8 MINUTES COOKING TIME 10 MINUTES

INGREDIENTS
10-15 Blueberries

1Banana

½ Avocados

Coffee powder (optional)

2 tsp. Milk powder
½ cup milk

INSTRUCTIONS

1. Peel the bananas and chop them roughly and add them in blender.
2. Add blueberries into the blender leaving 2 for garnishing, and add avocado as well.
3. Add rest of the ingredients and blend the contents well.
4. The smoothie so formed should have the consistency of thick to medium.
5. Pour the smoothie and garnish it with blueberries on the top.

It's fresh, It's fulfilling, it's HEALTHY!

DESSERT 6
PEAR IN CARAMEL
NUTRITIONAL VALUE 62.3 Cal PROTEIN 0.2g FAT 1.1 g
CARBOHYDRATES 14.2g

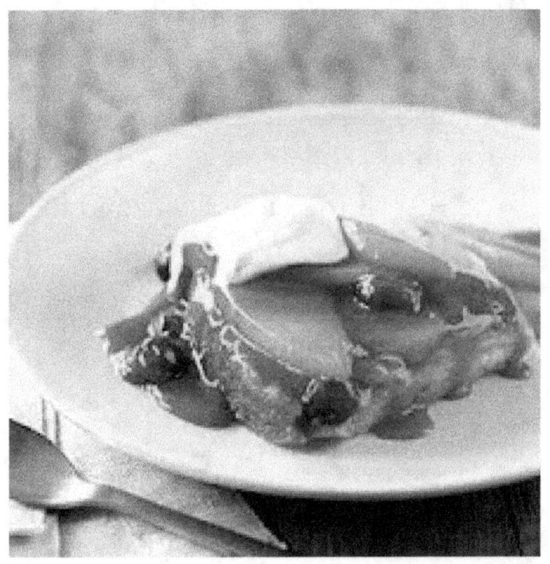

INGREDIENTS

1. 4 tablespoons butter

2. 1/2 cup sour cream

3. 2 cup packed dark brown sugar

4. 1/4 cup coarsely chopped toasted pistachios

5. 4 pears, halved and cored

Preparation time: 25 minutes

INSTRUCTIONS

1. Preheat the oven to 400 degrees. Add butter to a baking pan. Heat until it melts. Drizzle sugar over the butter; add pears. Bake until tender.

2. Remove from oven; turn over the pears and garnish with pan sauce. Get back to oven, bake for about 10 more minutes.

3. Allow it to cool down. Top pears with handful of sour cream, sprinkle with caramel pan sauce, drizzle nuts and serve.

BREAKFAST 7
KALE AND SPINACH SMOOTHIE

NUTRITIONAL VALUE 38 Cal PROTEIN 1g FAT 0 g
CARBOHYDRATES 9g

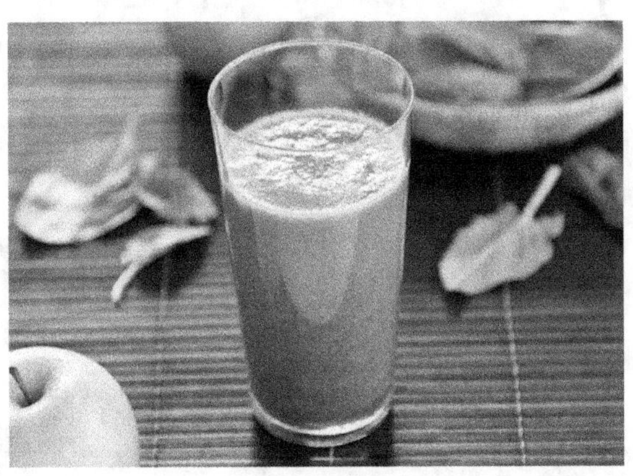

Greens serve a high source of vitamins and Iron. Kale and spinach are just the same. Smoothie for breakfast is a marvelous option for paleo diet practitioners.

SERVES 2 PREPARATION TIME 7 MINUTES COOKING TIME 0 MINUTES

INGREDIENTS

Kale- 200 gms

Spinach- 400 gms

Water (optional)

Ice (optional)

INSTRUCTIONS

1. Roughly tear the kale and spinach leaves and add them to the blender. Blend it well, and keep the consistency from medium to thick.

2. Add water if you want to keep it a little less dense or add ice if you want a freezer kind of drink.

Add this smoothie as a part of the breakfast as it not only provides a kick start to your day but serves as a great option for post work out drinks.

LUNCH 7
CHICKEN AND CABBAGE SALAD
NUTRITIONAL VALUE 339 Cal PROTEIN 28g FAT 8 g
CARBOHYDRATES 37g

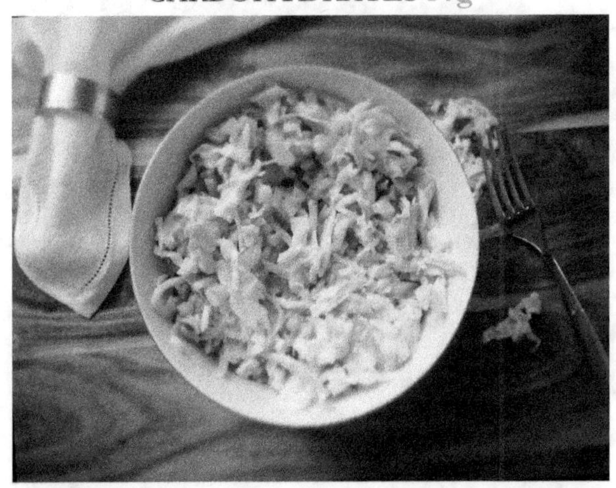

For those days when you really want to cook their heart out and go for a heavier option than just lighter salads for lunch , go for this creamy chicken recipe !

SERVES 2 TOTAL TIME 30 MINUTES
INGREDIENTS
½ shredded green cabbage

1 chicken breast, boneless and skinless

½ tsp. olive oil

½ cup avocado oil

½ large shallot

3 cloves garlic, chopped

½ tablespoon lime juice

½ tablespoon fish sauce

½ tablespoon salt

¼ teaspoon white pepper

½ teaspoon sugar, coconut palm
½ teaspoon apple cider vinegar
1-2 small carrots
1 thinly sliced spicy red chile pepper
Handful cilantro leaves
Handful mint leaves

INSTRUCTIONS

1. Take a large ball and place the shredded cabbage inside it.
2. This bowl needs to be filled with cold water.
3. Add little bit of salt to it and stir to combine. Set it and let marinate for 20 minutes.
4. While the cabbage is soaking in the water, grill the chicken. Carfully rub the chicken breast all over using olive oil. Dress with a bit of salt and pepper according to taste.
5. Add the chicken on the hot grill and let it cook for about 6 minutes, flipping every couple of minutes.
6. Get ready with a bowl of ice water and shift the cooked chicken to equip it for the ice water bath. Set it aside to be cooled for at least 5 minutes.
7. While the chicken is again busy soaking, you can heat the avocado oil in a pan over high heat. Now, bring the shallots and boil until they turn translucent, for at least 2 minutes. Add the garlic.

8. Stir-fry the recipe until it attains a golden color, while stirring regularly to evade scorching, for nearly 3 more minutes.

9. Add the oil into a medium sized bowl via a strainer, while catching the shallots and garlic to drain; save the oil and allow it to cool for 5 minutes.

10. When the oil gets enough cool, mix it together with the lime juice, salt, fish sauce, white pepper, apple cider vinegar, coconut palm sugar to make the dressing.

11. Shred the chicken together with the grain, by making use of the forks, and setting them aside.

12. Remove the cabbage and let it dry with paper towels.

13. In a large bowl, mix the chicken, cabbage, carrots, cilantro, chile pepper, mint, and the salad dressing.

14. Toss the ingredients to combine. Add salt according to taste, then serve topped with the fried shallots and garlic.

This is a smart salad which pleases most of the people following paleo diets. A little tricky to conduct the procedure but a tasty dish awaits behind all that hard work.

TUNA AND TOMATO BURGERS

NUTRITIONAL VALUE 150 Cal PROTEIN 18g FAT 7g
CARBOHYDRATES 4g

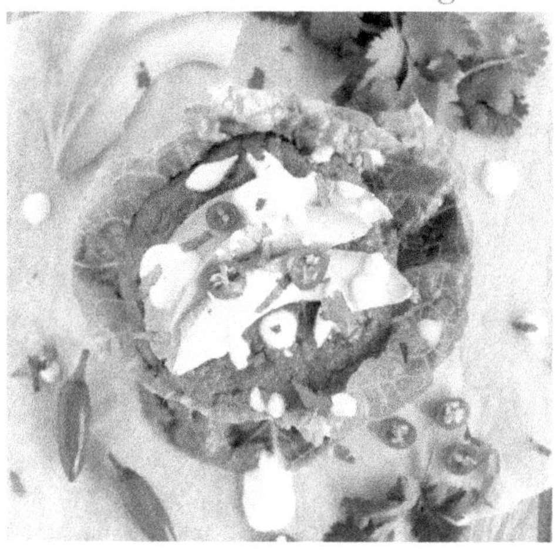

Burgers for dinner? Yes! Burgers for dinner!

Being paleo should never stop you from being interesting and trying out various forms of other dishes, such as this amazing burger, learn how to make this!

INGREDIENTS

2 cup of tuna, drained and rinsed
2 red onion, finely chopped
2 red chili, finely chopped
1 crushed garlic clove
2 eggs
4 tbsp of tomato paste
1 tbsp of coconut flour
Salt and pepper to taste

For serving

Burger buns
Lettuce
Avocado
Extra chilli
Fresh coriander (cilantro)
Greek yoghurt

INSTRUCTIONS

1. Heat your oven in advance at 175'C (350'F).

2. Line a baking sheet parchment paper and set aside.

3. Keep your burger's ingredients into a medium-large sized bowl and stir well till they are nicely combined.

4. Carefully roll and flatten the tuna mixture using your hands into 6, even sized burger Pattie. Finally place them on your baking tray.

5. Add in the microwave and cook for the next 10 minutes.

6. Serve immediately.

This meal might not be as low carb as paleo diets focus on but certainly is the best way to have as cheat meals without cheating whole with the paleo routine!

DESSERT 7
JAM ZUCCHINI
NUTRITIONAL VALUE 30 Cal PROTEIN 0g FAT 0g
CARBOHYDRATES 7g

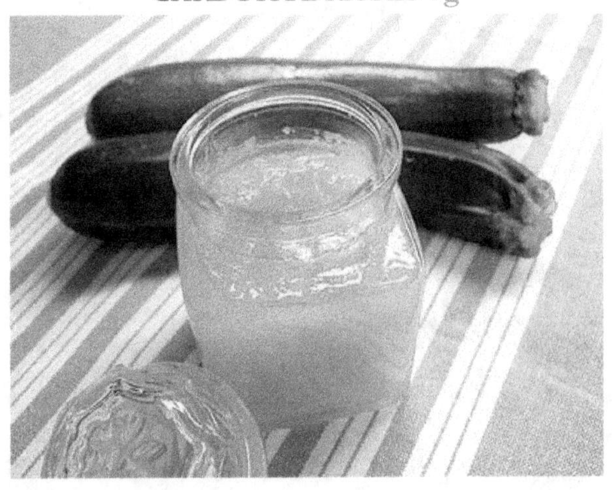

INGREDIENTS

6 cups of grated zucchini (peeled)

$\frac{1}{2}$ cup water

6 cups sugar

$\frac{1}{3}$ cup lemon juice

1(20 ounce) can crushed pineapple in juice

1(6 ounce) box cherry Jell-O

1(2 ounce) fruit pectin

Preparation time: 20 minutes

1. Prepare 5 glass pint jars, and add them to an oven with a cookie sheet on 200 degrees. In a pan, boil ½ cup of water and zucchini.

2. Bring 1/2 cup water and 6 cups of zucchini to a boil and allow them to simmer for 5 minutes.

3. Add lemon juice, sugar, and pineapple; boil for 5 minutes.

4. Stir in the jello; boil for another 2 minutes.

5. Remove from heat and move your pot towards a cool burner, taking out the jars from the oven, pour out water and scoop mixture into the hot jars.

BREAKFAST 8
BANANA NUT PORRIDGE

NUTRITIONAL VALUE 239 Cal PROTEIN 8g FAT 27g
CARBOHYDRATES 7g

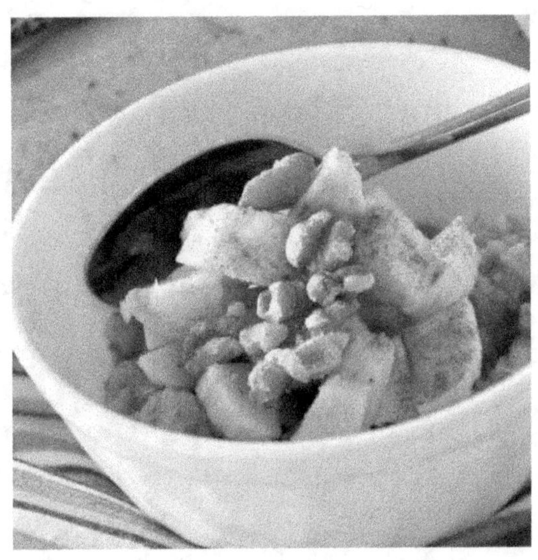

Porridge is one amongst that ultimate form of breakfast, after oats. Give it a banana spin to your normal porridge making it healthier and team it with nuts!

INGREDIENTS

¼ cup cashews, raw

¼ cup almonds, raw

¼ cup pecans, raw

1 ripe banana

1 cup of coconut milk

1 tsp cinnamon

Dash of sea salt to soak water

INSTRUCTIONS

1. Add the nuts in a large-sized bowl and drizzle the sea salt over them. Fill up the bowl with the filtered water to make sure that the nuts are covered by minimum 1 inch of water. Cover it thoroughly and soak throughout the night.
2. Drain off the nuts and wash for 2 or 3 times, till the water runs clear.
3. Bring the drained nuts within a high speed blender or a food processor. Mix the nuts together with the coconut milk, banana, and cinnamon until the mixture becomes smooth.
4. Distribute the ingredients among the bowl and let it microwave for nearly 40 seconds.
5. Serve with chopped nuts, raisins and an extra splash of milk if desired.

Rich with nutrients and warm flavors, but unfortunately a little less liked by kids, add waffles with this porridge recipe to have the perfect breakfast!

LUNCH 8
CHICKEN TACO SALAD
NUTRITIONAL VALUE 310 Cal PROTEIN 25g FAT 13g
CARBOHYDRATES 22g

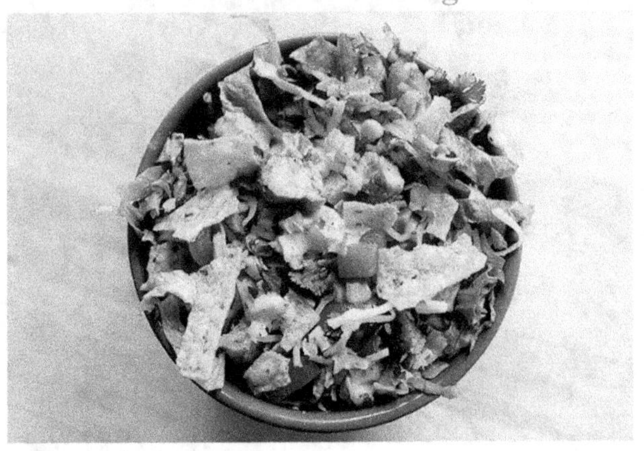

This lunch recipe couldn't have met a simpler and more convenient fate. Made from the wholesome and delicious ingredients, these paleo chicken taco salad is best eaten fresh, so get set for this health-studded paradise.

INGREDIENTS
2 boneless and skinless chicken breasts

2 cups of romaine lettuce

1 diced tomato;

½ diced avocado

½ diced bell pepper

¼ cup of mayonnaise, homemade

2 tbsp of olive oil;

2 tbsp of lime juice;

¼ cup finely chopped cilantro

For taco seasoning

- 1 tbsp of chili powder
- ¼ tsp of garlic powder;
- 1 tsp of ground cumin;
- ¼ tsp of onion powder;
- ¼ tsp of red pepper flakes;
- ¼ tsp of oregano;
- ¼ tsp of paprika;
- Sea salt to taste
- Freshly ground black pepper to taste

INSTRUCTIONS

1. Get the grill ready by pre-heating at medium-high.
2. Mix the taco-seasoning ingredients together in a bowl.
3. Stroke the chicken using half of the taco seasoning.
4. Add the chicken to the preheated grill.
5. Cook the chicken for 10 to 12 minutes, turning if needed.
6. Let the chicken cool down and then cut it into cubes.
7. Add the mayo, olive oil, lime juice, and the other half of the taco seasoning in a small bowl.

8. Use a large sized bowl to toss the tomatoes, lettuce, and avocado.

9. Dress the salad using the chicken and sprinkle dressing on top.

10. Serve with cilantro topped.

The lettuce, tomatoes, avocado and bell pepper add vibrancy and show off the nutrients within this colorful salad. For picky eaters you can add the contents into separate bowl.

SKINNY STRAWBERRY CAKE SMOOTHIE

NUTRITIONAL VALUE 230 Cal PROTEIN 3g FAT 13g
CARBOHYDRATES 25g

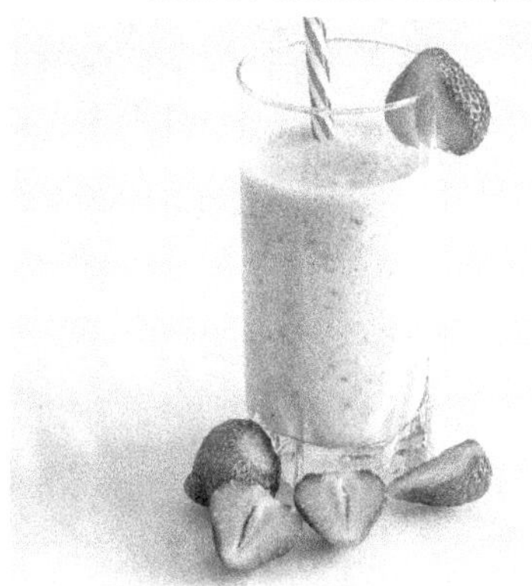

An easy and convenient to make smoothie, the strawberry paleo cake is not only healthy but also tastes like dessert! A great way to energize yourself during the noon & sneak in to a serving of fruit!

INGREDIENTS

200 grams of strawberries, unsweetened and frozen
180mL of milk, non-fat or non-dairy
5mL of butter extract
Sweetener or Truvia, to taste (Optional)

INSTRUCTIONS

1. Combine all the ingredients within a blender in the same order they are listed in.
2. Pulse the mixture until it gets smooth.
3. Serve and drink immediately.

Note: **Any milk may work for you, be it** 1%, 2%, soy or almond milk.

Additionally if you don't have butter extract, you may use the vanilla extract instead.

BAKED SALMON WITH ROASTED BEETS AND ASPARAGUS

NUTRITIONAL VALUE 303.4 Cal PROTEIN 11g FAT 18g
CARBOHYDRATES 25g

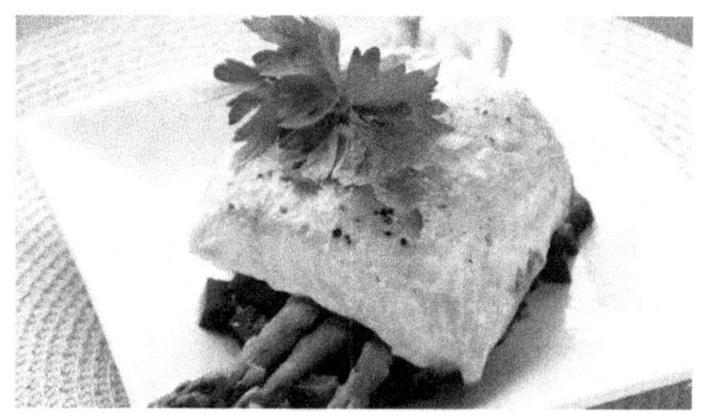

Asparagus and beets are two veggies that work amazingly well with the salmon. This simple yet convenient dish provides you with the leverage to be served with any fresh vegetable or fish.

SERVES 4 PREPARATION TIME 10 MINUTES
COOKING TIME 15 MINUTES

INGREDIENTS

4 wild and fresh salmon fillets;

4 tbsp coconut oil or butter;

4 tsp dill, chopped

14 sprigs of asparagus, fresh and hard base taken off;

4 red beets, chopped in cubes;

Salt and pepper for taste;

4 pieces of the heavy duty foil;

INSTRUCTIONS

1. Heat your oven in advance at 500 F.
2. Keep a bed of 4 asparagus and beet cubes on each of the four pieces of the foil, followed by topping with the salmon fillet.
3. Add 1 tbsp of dill and butter on top of each salmon fillet and close the foil by folding the top, followed by pinching and folding the sides to form a compact sized pocket to ensure no stream escapes.
4. Bake for 10 minutes in the hot oven.
5. Ensure checking on the fish regularly so it doesn't get overcooked.
6. Serve topped with your favourite herbs.

This meal might not only focus on low carb diet, but is also the best way to have a cheat meal without cheating on your paleo-diet routine. So, embrace yourself and gift yourself this dinner and have a great evening.

BANANA CUPCAKE

NUTRITIONAL VALUE 226 Cal PROTEIN 3g FAT 9.6 g
CARBOHYDRATES 32.6 g

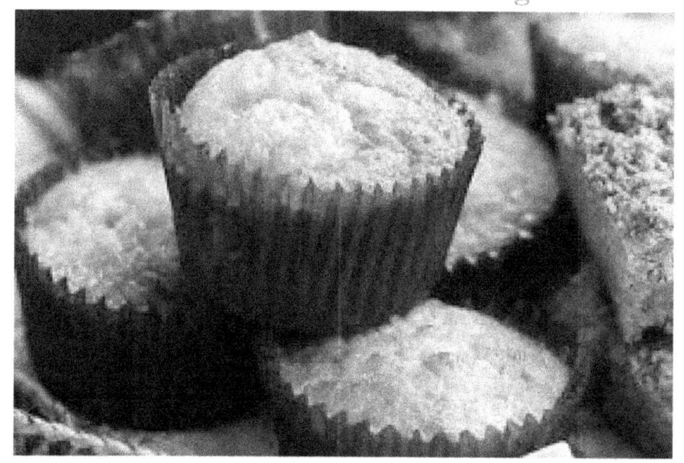

INGREDIENTS

3 bananas, mashed

2 teaspoons baking soda

1 cup white sugar

3 tablespoons buttermilk

2 eggs, lightly beaten

1 cup chopped pecans

3/4 cup vegetable oil

1 cup confectioners' sugar

2 cups all-purpose flour

Preparation time: 35 minutes

1. Preheat oven to 300 degrees F. Also, grease 14 muffin cups.
2. In a medium bowl, beat white sugar and bananas until smooth; add eggs, one after the other, until well incorporated. Stir in vegetable oil and blend for 2 minutes. Stir in buttermilk, baking soda and flour; mix well. Pour this batter into the prepared muffin cups.
3. Now, bake the muffin cups until you could cleanly take out a toothpick inserted out of a cupcake, after 20 to 30 minutes.

COCONUT CHICKEN FINGERS

NUTRITIONAL VALUE 298 Cal PROTEIN 28g FAT 12 g
CARBOHYDRATES 0 g

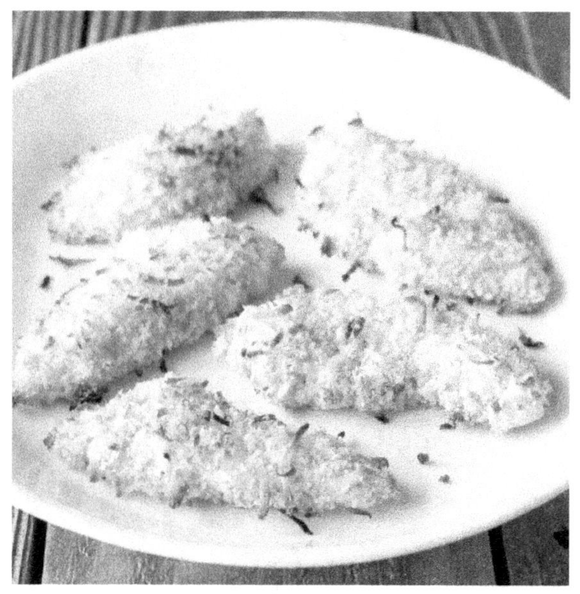

Chicken tenders are Paleo and Gluten free in nature and are easy and quick meal to make. We recommend you to double the recipe and heat them again and again throughout the entire week for extra fast dinners.

SERVES 4 PREPARATION TIME 5 MINUTES
COOKING TIME 20 MINUTES

INGREDIENTS

1 pound of skinless and boneless chicken tenders

1 egg

½ cup of cashew flour

1 cup coconut, unsweetened and shredded

¼ tsp salt for taste

¼ pepper for taste

¼ tsp garlic powder

¼ tsp cinnamon

INSTRUCTIONS

1. Heat the oven in advance at 375 degrees.
2. Whisk the eggs in a large bowl and set them aside.
3. Mix coconut, cashew flour and spices in a different dish or a bowl.
4. Lightly dip each chicken tender/finger in the whisked egg followed by dipping in the batter
5. Take a baking sheet lined with a parchment paper and keep the coated chicken tenders on it.
6. Next, bake for at least 15 minutes or until the tenders get golden brown in color and there's no pink on the inside.

The combination of chicken fingers and coconut makes a great breakfast and sure to be your secret best friends. In fact the combination has a great potential to make you fall in love with it. The recipe is quite easy and convenient to prepare and doesn't require anything else to be a complete meal.

GLUTTEN-FREE EGG ROLL IN BOWL

NUTRITIONAL VALUE 200 Cal PROTEIN 8g FAT 1.5 g
CARBOHYDRATES 20 g

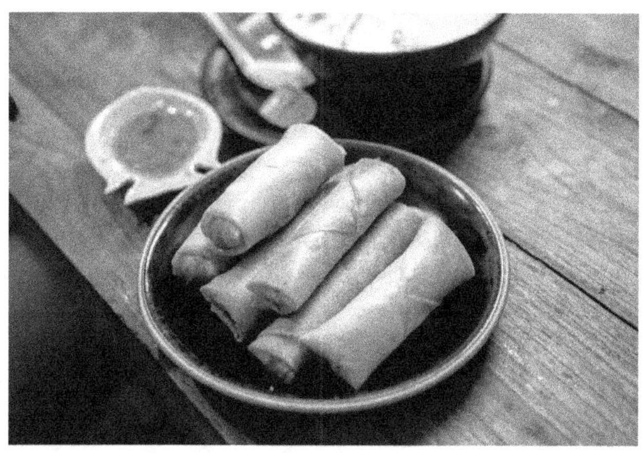

This meal not only focuses on low carb diet, but is also the best way to have a delicious meal without compromising on your paleo-diet routine. So, embrace yourself and start your afternoon with the egg roll in the bowl.

SERVES 12 PREPARATION TIME 15 MINUTES
COOKING TIME 25 MINUTES

INGREDIENTS

1 small cabbage head finely chopped into slices
2 medium carrots, chipped into long strips

1 tbsp coconut oil, unflavoured

½ cup of coconut aminos

1 ½ tbsp of the sesame oil

2 minced garlic cloves

3 diced green onions

1. Melt the unflavoured coconut oil at medium to high heat.
2. Add cabbage and the carrot.
3. Sautee until the mixture gets soft. Or else if it becomes extra dry, then add water and allow it to evaporate and soften the mixture.
4. Next, add in the sesame oil and the coconut aminos.
5. Keep boiling until it gets softer and the sauce is thoroughly absorbed.
6. Now, bring in the garlic and keep cooking until it gets fragrant.
7. Add the green onions at the top of the mixture.

This amazing paleo egg roll in a bowl has earned itself the reputation of bringing huge smiles on faces, so no matter if you have to throw a house party to your loved ones or a little bash with your partner, this Paleo recipe will never disappoint you.

CARAMALIZED ONION AVOCADO BURGERS

NUTRITIONAL VALUE 324 Cal PROTEIN 13g FAT 11 g
CARBOHYDRATES 48 g

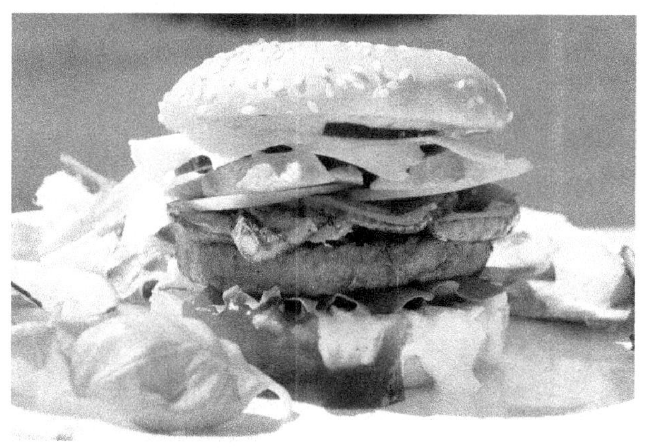

Whoever says burgers can't be paleo or healthy, haven't come across this magical avocado burger. Served on a slice of tomato topped aesthetically with Caramelized Onions, it will make you a big fan of its recipe. A quick and convenient meal ready within half an hour, this will keep your family on repeat!

SERVES 6 PREPARATION TIME 5 MINUTES
COOKING TIME 25 MINUTES

1 pound: Ground beef {This makes 6 burgers of ¼lb each}
1 tsp of salt, pepper to taste
1 tsp garlic powder
2 tsp coconut oil
2 thinly sliced onions
2 ½ tbsp of balsamic vinegar
1 beef steak tomato finely sliced into 6 thick pieces
1 ½ cups of green leaf lettuce, finely shredded
3 avocados

INSTRUCTIONS

1. First and the foremost, bring a medium skillet to boil over medium high heat.
2. Add 1 tsp of coconut oil, and once it melts, add in the thinly sliced onions. Next, Sauté till the mixture gets lightly caramelized in color, while stirring it occasionally. {for at least 10 minutes}
3. Bring in the balsamic vinegar and sauté the mixture for the next 5 minutes while stirring occasionally. Set it aside.

For Burgers:

1. Make six ¼ lb. burgers using the ground beef.

2. Season both the sides of the burger using garlic powder, salt and pepper.
3. Next, heat a large sized skillet to medium-high heat. Add the remaining 1 tsp of the coconut oil.
4. Keep the burgers in the skillet while sauting each side for atleast 2 minutes.
5. Take away from the skillet and let it cool for a minute.
6. Align the burgers.
7. Cautiously place 1 large slice of the tomato on a plate and dress with the shredded lettuce, the burger itself, 2 tbsp of the caramelized onions, and lastly top it with the avocado you sliced.
8. Serve with mustard (gluten-free).

The rich blend of beef, onions and tomatoes not only provides a treat to your taste buds but also takes this recipe to the height of amaze. These avocado burgers make a perfectly healthy treat this fall.

DINNER 9

BROCCOLI & BEEF RECIPE

NUTRITIONAL VALUE 178 Cal PROTEIN 19.2g FAT 3 g
CARBOHYDRATES 19 g

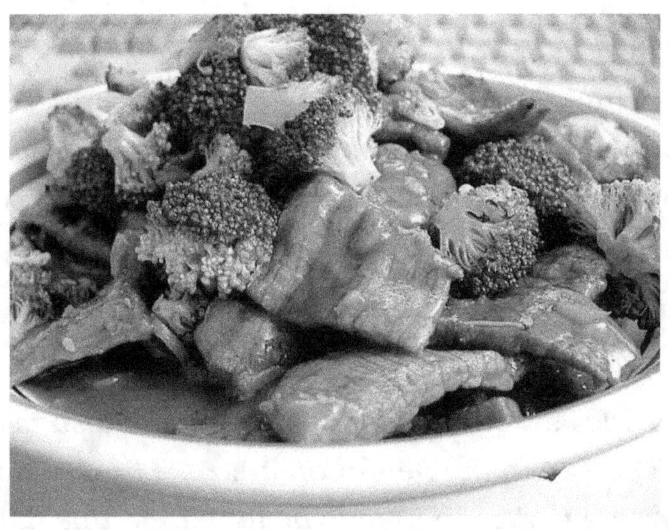

The beef and broccoli you are served in restaurants is delicious but too heavy and salty. This ditto recipe fixes that by making it Paleo friendly without losing the main flavors.

SERVES 2 PREPARATION TIME 5 MINUTES
COOKING TIME 15 MINUTES

INGREDIENTS

2 cups broccoli florets

1/2 lb beef, sliced thin and precooked
3 precooked garlic cloves crushed or simply use the garlic
powder
1 tsp gingers freshly grated or simply use the ginger
powder
2 tbsp coconut aminnos or use tamari sauce, to taste
Coconut oil (for cooking)

INSTRUCTIONS

1. Add 2 tbsp of coconut oil into a saucepan or skillet and heat over medium-high heat.

2. Next, add the broccoli florets into the saucepan.

3. When broccoli florets soften to the desired level, add in the beef.

4. Boil the mixture for 2 minutes and bring in the ginger, garlic and coconut aminos/tamari sauce.

5. Serve immediately.

This meal might not only focus on low carb diet, but is also the best way to have a cheat meal without cheating on your paleo-diet routine. So, embrace yourself and gift yourself this dinner broccoli and beef.

DESSERT 9

SWEET RICE PUDDING

NUTRITIONAL VALUE 324 Cal PROTEIN 13g FAT 11 g
CARBOHYDRATES 48 g

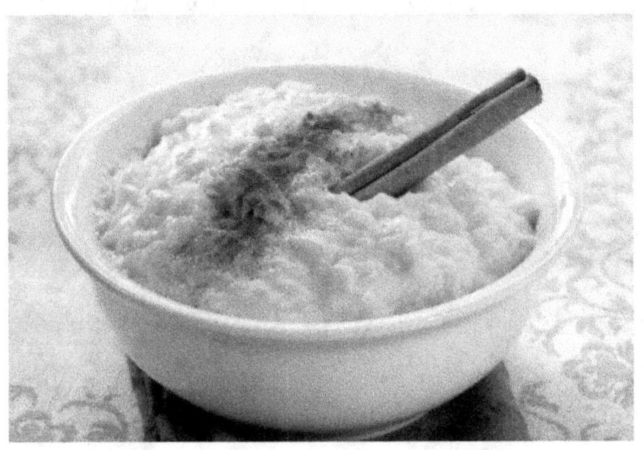

INGREDIENTS

1. 1 ½ cups cooked rice
2. ¼ cup raisins
3. 2 eggs
4. 1 ½ cups milk
5. ½ cup sugar
6. ½ teaspoon ground nutmeg
7. Additional milk

Preparation time: 55 minutes

INSTRUCTIONS

1. In a greased casserole, add raisins and rice.
   Simultaneously, whisk sugar, eggs, nutmeg; and
   pour over the rice.
2. Bake the mixture in preheated oven, at 375° for an
   hour. Allow it to cool. If needed, you could also
   pour milk over each serving.

BREAKFAST 10

QUICK AND EASY BREAKFAST SCRAMBLE

NUTRITIONAL VALUE 199.3 Cal PROTEIN 13g FAT 15 g
CARBOHYDRATES 2 g

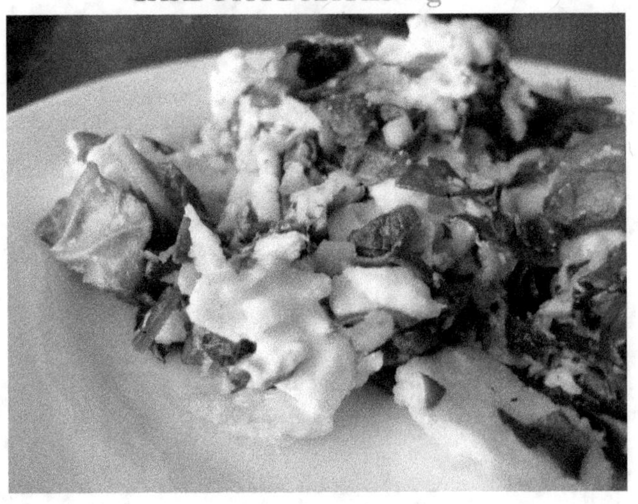

What makes this marvelously elaborate recipe a pure treat is its gluten-free nature. Get ready with your muffin try, as this good morning recipe is not only easy to prepare and amazing to eat, but also makes a perfect breakfast idea if you were ever to throw a treat to a crowd!

SERVES 1 PREPARATION TIME 10 MINUTES
COOKING TIME 10 MINUTES

INGREDIENTS

3 whisked eggs

4 mushrooms (baby bella)

1/3 cup of the red- peppers

½ cup spinach

Deli ham, 2 slices

1 tbsp ghee or coconut oil
Salt and pepper to taste

INSTRUCTIONS

1. Chop the vegetables and the ham together.

2. Keep ½ tbsp of butter into a frying pan and allow it to melt. Sauté the hams and vegetables together.

3. Take a separate frying pan and add the whisked eggs and ½ tbsp of butter.

4. Allow this mixture to be cooked on medium-high heat while stirring for in order to prevent overcooking.

5. When the eggs are cooked thoroughly, season them with pepper and salt accordingly.

6. Last but not the least, combine the saute'd vegetables and ham with the egg mix.

7. Serve immediately.

Quick and easy breakfast scramble is paleo in nature and is easy and quick meal to make. We recommend you to double the delight of the recipe by sharing it with your loved ones as a great breakfast.

GOOD NOON CHICKEN BURRITO BOWLS

NUTRITIONAL VALUE 350 Cal PROTEIN 14 g FAT 11 g
CARBOHYDRATES 42 g

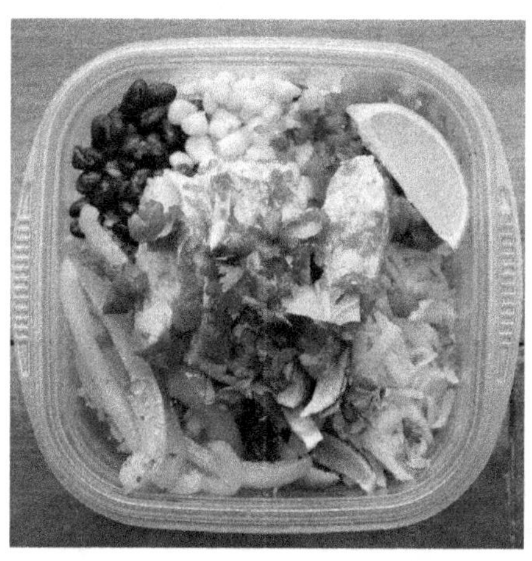

This good noon chicken burrito bowls not only focuses on low carb diet, but is also serves the pinnacle of delight to your taste buds. So, sit back and relax, your afternoon is all set to be enlightened by this burrito bowl.

SERVES 4 PREPARATION TIME 10 MINUTES
COOKING TIME 20 MINUTES

INGREDIENTS

2 cups of kale
1 ½ cups of grape tomatoes

3 cups of cubed or shredded chicken

¾ cup of canned corn

2 cups of canned black beans

1 cup of cooked rice

1 ½ tsp paprika

½ tsp of cumin

1/3 tsp of cayenne

1/3 tsp pepper

INSTRUCTIONS

1. Follow the directions to prepare rice or you could purchase the cooked rice as well.
2. Mix the rice in cumin, paprika, cayenne, and pepper and let them cook with rice for about 5 minutes.
3. Coat the container or the bowl to be used with tomatoes, kale, rice, corn and beans.
4. You are ready to serve.

This amazing burrito bowl has long known for pleasing the crowd, so no matter if you have to throw a house party to your loved ones or a little bash with your partner, this Paleo recipe will never disappoint you.

DESSERT 10

NUTRITIONAL VALUE 53 Cal PROTEIN 0.3 g FAT 11 g
CARBOHYDRATES 3 g

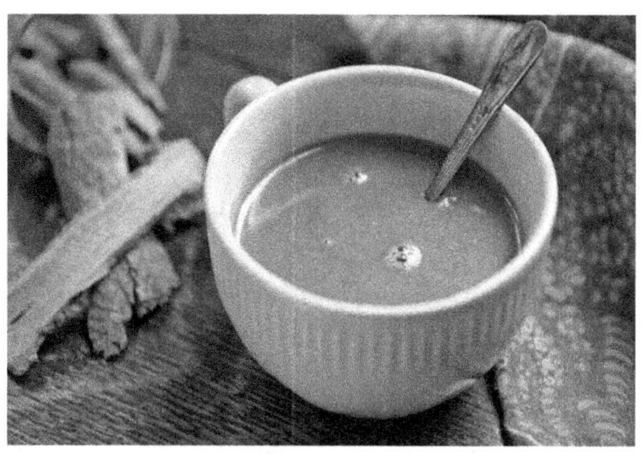

INGREDIENTS

4 cups milk

1/4 cup unsweetened cocoa powder

1/4 cup sugar

2 tsp. corn-starch

1 tsp. cinnamon

1/2 tsp. vanilla extract

1/4 tsp. chipotle powder

Pinch of nutmeg.

Pinch of cayenne

Preparation time: 10 minutes

INSTRUCTIONS

1. In a medium sauce pan, add all these ingredients.
2. Heat over medium-high heat until simmering while stirring frequently.
3. Remove from heat and serve.

PIZZA FRITTATA

NUTRITIONAL VALUE 314 Cal PROTEIN 23 g FAT 20 g
CARBOHYDRATES 11 g

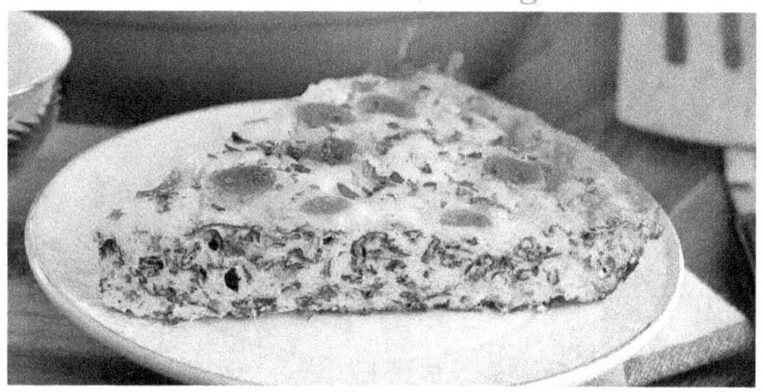

If you think pizza cannot be healthy then you are yet to come across this magician dish called the paleo pizza frittata. Served with the typical pizza sauce, it will soon take over the place of your favourite recipe.

SERVES 10 PREPARATION TIME 35 MINUTES
COOKING TIME 8 MINUTES

INGREDIENTS

½ pound Italian sausage
6 eggs
1 cup of pizza sauce

1/3 cup of fresh basil, worn out into small pieces
Pinch of salt, pepper and red pepper for taste
½ sliced green bell pepper
4 sliced button mushrooms
4 slices of pepperoni
2 cups of arugula
Fresh lemon juice from ½ lemons

INSTRUCTIONS

1. Heat the oven in advance at 350 degrees F.
2. Heat the skillet over medium-high heat.
3. Bring in the sausage while using a wooden spoon to divide it into smaller pieces, till there is no pink visible.
4. Deliberately layer the sausage across the skillet.
5. Turn down the heat to medium-low.
6. Take a large bowl; beat the eggs together with basil, salt, pepper, pizza sauce and red pepper flakes.
7. Add this mixture into skillet and allow it to cook in the pan for at least 5 minutes.
8. Dress the frittata using the mushrooms, green pepper slices, and pepperoni. Now, keep it in the oven and bake for 20 minutes.
9. Pitch arugula in olive oil and lemon and keep it on the top of frittata just before serving!

Just when you were bored of the typical lunch recipes, this frittata paved its way to our recipe book and came to your health and taste bud's rescue. Enjoy a

*rich blend of taste and health with this amazing
recipe and thank us later.*

139

DINNER 10
HEALTHY LIVER AND ONION DINNER

NUTRITIONAL VALUE 327.6 Cal PROTEIN 21 g FAT 15 g
CARBOHYDRATES 26 g

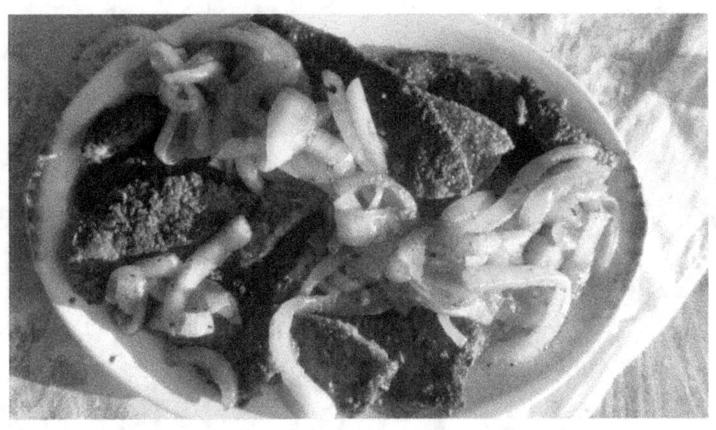

The combination of liver and onions make a great dinner and sure to be your secret best friends. In fact the combination has a great potential to make you love liver. The recipe is quite easy and convenient to prepare and doesn't require anything else to be a complete meal.

SERVES 4 PREPARATION TIME 10 MINUTES
COOKING TIME 25 MINUTES

INGREDIENTS

4 medium sized large slices of beef liver;

5 medium diced onions

6-7 tbsp butter;

Salt and pepper to taste;

1. Heat a saucepan or a skillet over medium to low heat and add 4 tbsp of butter and sliced onions.
2. Keep cooking slowly and gradually, while stirring often, for the next 20 minutes, or until the onions get really caramelized and soft.
3. Just 5 minutes before the onions are completely done; you could heat another pan on a medium-high heat and cook the beef liver using the remaining cooking fat, for a/bout 5 minutes on both the sides.
4. Serve the recipe topped with the tasty and creamy cooked onions.

The liver and onion you get from restaurants is delicious but too heavy and salty. This copycat recipe fixes that by making it healthy without losing the main flavors. It's also very quick and easy to make.

CONCLUSION